£19.95

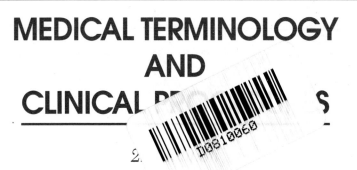

MEDICAL TERMINOLOGY
AND
CLINICAL ~~~~~ ~

MEDICAL TERMINOLOGY
AND
CLINICAL PROCEDURES

2nd Edition

Mary Bird SRN RN FAMS

Former Chief Examiner for AMSPAR (Medical Aspects)

MAGISTER CONSULTING LTD

Published in the UK by
Magister Consulting Ltd
Doral House
2b Manor Road
Kent BR3 5LE
UK

Copyright © 1999 Magister Consulting Ltd

First edition published 1995 by Publishing Initiatives (Europe) Ltd
Reprinted 1996, 1997
Second Edition 1999

Printed and bound in Great Britain by Redhouse Press Ltd

ISBN 1 873839 57 X

B–0048/2E(B–19)

CONTENTS

FOREWORD

The role of the foreword writer is to inform the reader what it is that makes the book in question special, and what separates it from others in the field. That being so, writing the foreword for this book does not present a challenge, for I know of no other book of this kind. The word 'unique' is frequently misused to mean only 'slightly different' from something else, whereas in fact it should define a total difference – a 'one-off', and Mary Bird's book is just that.

This is not a book one reads, it is a book that one *uses*. Those who purchase the book will find it will become indispensible, and well-worn! It is an essential guide and companion for anyone setting out on a medical career, whether as a medical secretary, practice manager, nurse or therapist. Within it are tools to make sense of any sort of medical discourse. Whether one is trying to understand a paper, text or a conversation on anything medical, then one should consult this guide.

In truth I am not sure where else to find such an eclectic mix of information; a dictionary may contain definitions, but this book goes further than that in many instances. Not long ago books such as this were deemed unfashionable, being strongly influenced by the 'medical model'. Nowadays I hope we have matured enough to acknowledge the worth and usefulness of guides like this, which do not set out to declaim, critique or analyse, but simply explain the words that medical professionals use.

I am full of admiration for the sort of writer who can carry out this expert task in the way that Mary Bird has here, for I cannot imagine even starting to compile a volume like this. I recommend it to you to use – it will be a good companion!

Sue Hinchliff

Head of Continuing Professional Development
Royal College of Nursing of the United Kingdom

ACKNOWLEDGEMENTS

This book is dedicated in grateful thanks to:

All my AMSPAR students, past and present, from whom I have learnt so much.

•

Olga de Souza, my predecessor as AMSPAR Chief Examiner, for her very high standards, which I have tried my best to maintain.

•

Michael, Susan, Ian, Beth and Iain, for all their support and encouragement, without which this book would never have been written!

•

And with love to my grandchildren James, Sarah, Jennifer and Christopher.

INTRODUCTION

This book is intended to provide an insight into medical terminology and the common clinical procedures met in the everyday work of health workers, including secretaries, receptionists, administrators and managers, as well as students in many other disciplines.

The breakdown of medical words into the basic prefixes, roots and suffixes, aims to help unravel the mystery of medical language and enable the reader to build a vast vocabulary in a surprisingly short time. Basic anatomy and physiology of the body have been included in order to provide further explanation and interest for the reader. Medical terms and abbreviations are grouped together with the appropriate body system, wherever possible; e.g. 'Angina pectoris' and 'Blood pressure' are explained in Section 5 - The Cardiovascular System.

At the end of each section are lists of abbreviations, terminology, diseases and disorders, and procedures and equipment related to that body system. The index at the end of the book contains the terms mentioned in the main text of each section, and not all of those contained in these lists.

Sections on drugs and preventive medicine, including immunisation schedules and Notifiable Diseases are included. Areas concerning the work of the pathology and X-ray departments are intended to provide more knowledge of the principles of common tests performed on patients.

At the outset of my career, I was encouraged always to remember that the welfare of the patient was the priority. I express the hope that this book, by giving a better understanding, will enable all those involved in patient care to deal more effectively with that most important person - the patient!

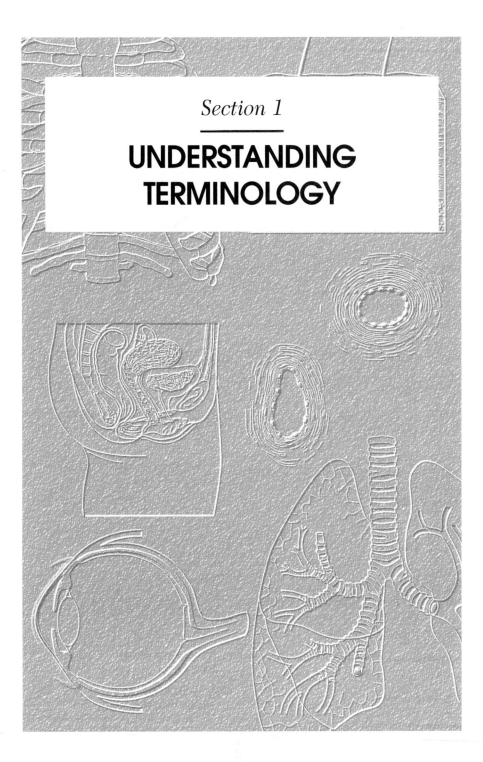

Section 1

UNDERSTANDING
TERMINOLOGY

THE ORIGIN AND CONSTRUCTION OF MEDICAL TERMS

To the uninitiated, medical terms can seem frightening and unintelligible. As with any speciality, a language has developed which separates those 'within' from outsiders, conveying a mystique which appears hard to penetrate. However, it is necessary to have a precise language to describe a medical condition or procedure, in order that other members of the medical profession may accurately interpret diagnoses etc. Most medical words are derived from Greek and Latin sources - international languages until the eighteenth century. Some Arabic, Anglo-Saxon and German origins are also involved. By understanding and following some basic rules, the mystery of medical terminology can be revealed.

BASIC CONSTRUCTION OF MEDICAL TERMS

Medical terms consist of the following parts:
- a **prefix**,
- a **root or stem**,
- a **suffix**,
- a **combining vowel**.

Prefix

This part of the word is found before the stem and qualifies, i.e. tells us more about, the stem.

e.g. **poly** - meaning 'many'.

Not all words have a prefix.

Root or stem

This is the main part of the word, which gives the information about that which is being described.

e.g. **neur** - meaning 'nerve'.

Suffix

This part of the word is found following the stem and gives further information about the stem.

e.g. **-itis** - meaning 'inflammation of'.

All medical terms have a suffix.

Prefix	Root/stem	Suffix
poly /	neur /	itis

Combining vowel

This is a vowel which is added to the stem, when necessary, to allow easy pronunciation; it is usu-

ally an 'o'. If the suffix begins with a vowel then it is not required.

e.g. **poly/neur/itis** meaning 'inflammation of many nerves'.

Some further examples

En/cephal/o/gram means 'a recording of brain waves'.

As there is no vowel in the suffix, o is inserted between the stem and suffix.

en- is a prefix meaning 'within'.

-cephal- is a stem meaning 'head', i.e. the brain.

-gram is a suffix meaning 'a tracing or writing'.

Peri/card/itis meaning 'inflammation of the pericardium' (the layer of tissue around the heart).

peri- is a prefix meaning 'around'.

-cardi- is a stem meaning 'heart'.

-itis is a suffix meaning 'inflammation'.

However, there is a vowel at the end of the stem 'cardi' as well as a vowel 'i' at the beginning of 'itis'. One of the 'i's is dropped to form the word 'pericarditis'. No added 'o' is necessary.

The letter 'h' is also treated as a vowel sound and is dropped when combining with another vowel, or where the pronunciation would be clumsy:

An/aem/ia literally means 'lack of blood', but in medical terms it is the reduction of red cells or haemoglobin content in the blood.

an- is a prefix meaning 'absence of'.

-haem- is a stem meaning 'blood'.

-ia is a suffix meaning 'condition of'.

The 'h' of the stem is dropped as 'anhaemia' is difficult to pronounce.

Leuc/o/rrhoea meaning 'white discharge'.

leuc- is a stem meaning 'white'.

-o- is a combining vowel added to the stem.

-rrhoea is a suffix meaning 'running or discharge'.

By following the rules illustrated above, many terms can be understood or constructed.

The following are some examples:

COMMON PREFIXES

a- or **an-**	meaning absence of
anti-	meaning against

ante-	meaning before
dys-	meaning difficult/abnormal/ painful
endo-	meaning inside
haemo-	meaning blood
hypo-	meaning under/low
hyper-	meaning above/high

COMMON SUFFIXES

Surgical procedures

-otomy – meaning cutting into or dividing
osteotomy meaning cutting into bone

-ostomy – meaning making an artificial opening
tracheostomy meaning making an artificial opening into the trachea

N.B. Note the difference between **tracheotomy** and **tracheostomy**. In a **tracheostomy** the hole is left open, whereas a tracheotomy is a simple cutting into and then closing.

-orrhaphy means a sewing or repair
herniorrhaphy meaning repair of a hernia

-ectomy means surgical removal
appendicectomy meaning surgical removal of the appendix

-pexy meaning fixation
orchiopexy meaning fixation of an unde-scended testicle

Other surgical and procedure suffixes

-oscopy	meaning examination with a lighted instrument
-plasty	meaning reshape or form
-tripsy	meaning crushing
-centesis	meaning puncturing and drawing off (tapping)
-gram	meaning record/picture
-graph	meaning instrument that records
-graphy	meaning procedure of recording
-opsy	meaning looking at
-stasis	meaning stopping
-clasis	meaning breaking

Other important suffixes

-ia, -iasis, -osis, -ism	all meaning condition of
-itis	meaning inflammation of
-pathy	meaning disease of
-genic	meaning produced from or originating from

-al, -ic, -iac	meaning pertaining to
-oid	meaning shape or form
-ology	meaning scientific study of
-cyte	meaning cell

COMMON ROOTS OR STEMS

(see *Figures 1* and *2*)

The following is a list of common roots or stems together with a combining vowel. Some have two different stems, one from the Greek and one from the Latin, e.g. **phleb/o** (Greek) and **ven/o** (Latin) both meaning 'vein'.

STEM	MEANING
Abdomin/o - Lapar/o	abdomen
Aden/o	gland
An/o	anus
Andr/o	man
Angi/o - Vas/o	vessel
Appendic/o	appendix
Arteri/o	artery
Arthr/o	joint
Aur/i - Ot/o	ear
Bronch/o	bronchus
Bronchiol/o	bronchiole (small termination of bronchial tubes)
Cardi/o	heart
Cephal/o	head
Cerebr/o	cerebrum (part of brain)
Cheil/o	lip
Cheir/o	hand/surgery
Cholecyst/o	gallbladder
Choledoch/o	common bile duct
Chondr/o	cartilage
Col/o	colon (large intestine)
Cost/o	rib
Crani/o	cranium (skull containing brain)
Cyst/o	bladder
Dent/o - Odont/o	tooth
Derm/o - Dermat/o	skin
Duoden/o	duodenum (part of small intestine)
Encephal/o	brain
Gastr/o	stomach
Gingiv/o	gums
Gloss/o - Lingu/o	tongue
Gynaec/o	woman
Hep/o - Hepat/o	liver
Hyster/o - Metr/o - Uter/o	womb/uterus

Ile/o	ileum (part of small intestine)
Ili/o	ilium (bone of pelvis)
Irid/o	iris (of eye)
Kerat/o	cornea of eye
Lacrim/o	tear
Lamina	part of vertebra
Lob/o	lobe (e.g. of lung)
Mast/o - Mamm/o	breast
My/o - Myos	muscle
Myel/o	bone marrow/spinal cord
Myring/o - Tympan/o	eardrum
Nas/o - Rhin/o	nose
Nephr/o - Ren/o	kidney
Neur/o	nerve
Oesophag/o	oesophagus
Oophor/o	ovary
Ophthalm/o	eye
Orchi/o - Orchid/o	testicle/testis
Oste/o	bone
Pancreat/o	pancreas
Pharyng/o	pharynx
Phleb/o - Ven/o	vein
Phren/o	diaphragm
Pneumon/o - Pneum/o	lungs
Proct/o	rectum/anus
Prostat/o	prostate gland
Pyel/o	pelvis of kidney
Pylor/o	part of stomach
Rect/o	rectum
Sacr/o	sacrum (part of vertebrae)
Salping/o	fallopian tube
Sial/o	salivary gland
Splen/o	spleen
Spondyl/o - Vertebr/o	vertebra
Stomat/o	mouth
Ten/o - Tendin/o	tendon
Thorac/o - Steth/o	thorax (chest)
Thyr/o	thyroid gland
Trache/o	trachea (windpipe)
Trich/o	hair
Ureter/o	ureter (urinary system)
Urethr/o	urethra

LIST OF COMMON PREFIXES

The following is a list of common prefixes for combining with stems and suffixes.

PREFIX	MEANING
a- or an-	absence of, without
ab-	away from
acro-	extremity
ad-	towards
adipo-	fat
ambi-	both
amyl-	starch
ana-	up, excessive
aniso-	unequal
ante-	before
anti-	against
auto-	self
bi-	two
bili-	bile
bio-	life
brady-	slow
carpo-	wrist
centi-	hundred
chole-	bile
chrom-	colour
circum-	around
co-/con-	together with
contra-	against
cryo-	cold
crypto-	hidden
cyano-	blue
cyto-	cell
dacryo-	tear
dactyl-	finger
de-	away from/reversing
demi-	half
dextro-	to the right
di-	two
dia-	through
dys-	difficult, painful
ect-	without, outside
endo-	within, inside
epi-	upon
ery- erythro-	red
eu-	good, normal
ex-	out
extra-	outside
flavo-	yellow
gen-	referring to birth or producing
glyco-	sugar
haemo-	blood

4

hemi-	half	pleuro-	pleura, rib, side
hetero-	different, other	pneumo-	air
histo-	tissue	podo-	foot
homeo-	like	polio-	grey
homo-	same	poly-	many
hydro-	water, fluid	post-	after
hyper-	above, in excess of normal	pre-/pro-	before
		proto-	first
hypo-	below, under, less than normal	pseudo-	false
		psycho-	mind
iatro-	physician	pyo-	pus
idio-	peculiar to the individual	pyro-	fire, heat
		quadri-	four
in-	in	radio-	radiation
infra-	below	retro-	behind
inter-	between	steato-	fat
intra-	within	sub-	below
iso-	equal, same	supra-	above
karyo-	nucleus	syn-	with, union
kypho-	humped, rounded	tachy-	fast, rapid
lacto-	milk	tarso-	foot, eyelid
leuco-	white	teno-	tendon
lip/o	fat	tetra-	four
lympho-	lymphatic	thermo-	heat
macro-	large	thrombo-	blood clot
mal-	bad, abnormal	tox-/toxico-	poison
mega-	big, enlarged	tri-	three
melano-	black, dark, pigment	ultra-	beyond
meta-	beyond	uni-	one
metro-	measure, uterus	uro-	urine
micro-	small	vaso-	vessel
multi-	many	xantho-	yellow
myco-/myceto-	fungus	xero-	dry
narco-	stupor		

LIST OF COMMON SUFFIXES

		SUFFIX	MEANING
neo-	new	-aemia	blood
nocto- / nycto-	night	-aesthesia	sensibility
oligo-	scanty	-al	pertaining to
onycho-	nail	-algia	pain
oo-	egg, ovum	-an	pertaining to
oro-	mouth	-blast	immature cell
ortho-	straight	-cele	swelling/protrusion/ herniation
os-	opening, bone		
pachy-	thick	-centesis	puncture, drawing off
paedo-	child	-cide	killing, destroying
pan-	all	-cision	cutting
para-	alongside, close to	-clasis	breaking
patho-	disease	-coccus	round cell, type of bacteria
ped-	foot, child		
penta-	five	-cyte	cell
per-	through	-derm	skin
peri-	around	-desis	binding together
pharmaco-	drugs, chemist		
phren-	diaphragm		

-dynia	pain
-ectasis	dilatation
-ectomy	removal of
-form	having the formation or shape of
-genesis	forming or origin
-genic	producing or forming
-gram	a picture
-graph	a machine which records
-graphy	the procedure of recording
-iasis	condition of/state of
-iatric	pertaining to medicine/physician
-ism	condition of
-itis	inflammation of
-kinesis	movement, activity
-lith	stone
-lithiasis	condition of stones
-lysis	breaking down (keep splitting)
-malacia	softening
-megaly	enlargement
-meter	measure
-oid	likeness, resemblance
-ology	scientific study of
-oma	tumour
-opia	condition of the eye
-ose	sugar
-osis	condition of
-ostomy	making an opening (to remain)
-otomy	to cut into, divide
-ous	like, similar to
-paresis	weakness
-pathy	disease
-penia	lack of, decreased
-pexy	fixation of
-phage	eating, ingesting
-phagia	swallowing
-phasia	speech
-philia	loving, affinity for
-phobia	irrational fear of
-phylaxis	protection, prevention
-plasia	formation
-plasty	form, mould, reconstruct
-plegia	paralysis
-pnoea	breathing
-poiesis	making
-rhythmia	rhythm
-rrhage	to burst forth (heavy bleeding)
-rrhaphy	sewing, repair

-rrhexis	rupture of
-rrhoea	flowing, discharge
-sclerosis	hardening
-scope	lighted instrument used for examination
-scopy	examination with lighted instrument
-somatic	pertaining to the body
-stasis	cessation of movement/flow
-staxis	dripping (blood)
-stenosis	narrowing
-sthenia	strength
-taxia	co-ordination, order
-tome	cutting instrument
-tripsy	crushing of stones
-trophy	nourishment
-uria	condition of urine

COMMON PLURAL FORMS

The following rules apply when forming plural words:

SINGULAR ENDING	PLURAL ENDING
-us staphylococcus	**-i** staphylococci
-a vertebra	**-ae** vertebrae
-um atrium	**-a** atria
-is diagnosis	**-es** diagnoses
-oma stoma	**-omata** stomata
-ix cervix	**-ices** cervices
-ax thorax	**-aces** thoraces
-on ganglion	**-a** ganglia

AMERICANISMS

In American versions of medical terms, spellings are altered in the following ways. It is common to drop the silent double vowels (diphthong) as used in English spellings, e.g. 'ae' becomes 'e'.

The English stem 'haem', in American spelling is 'hem' (meaning blood).

Other examples are:

ENGLISH	AMERICAN
anaemia	anemia
anaesthesia	anesthesia
oedema	edema
dyspnoea	dyspnea

leucocyte   leukocyte
paediatric   pediatric

With the advent of word checks on computers, American style spellings of medical words is increasing in use. However, the English interpretation is used throughout this book.

ROOTS FOR BODY PARTS AND ORGANS

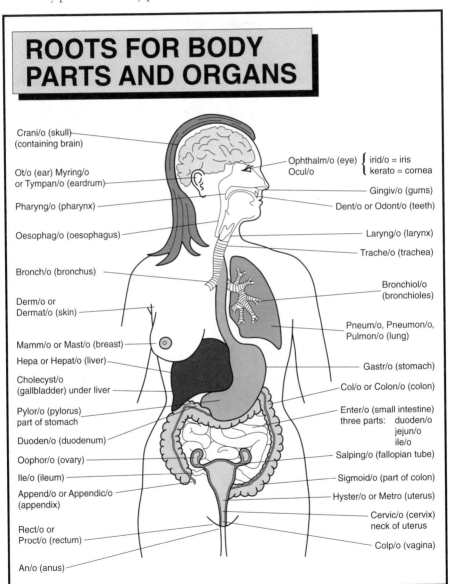

Crani/o (skull) (containing brain)

Ot/o (ear) Myring/o or Tympan/o (eardrum)

Pharyng/o (pharynx)

Oesophag/o (oesophagus)

Bronch/o (bronchus)

Derm/o or Dermat/o (skin)

Mamm/o or Mast/o (breast)

Hepa or Hepat/o (liver)

Cholecyst/o (gallbladder) under liver

Pylor/o (pylorus) part of stomach

Duoden/o (duodenum)

Oophor/o (ovary)

Ile/o (ileum)

Append/o or Appendic/o (appendix)

Rect/o or Proct/o (rectum)

An/o (anus)

Ophthalm/o (eye)   { irid/o = iris
Ocul/o   { kerato = cornea

Gingiv/o (gums)

Dent/o or Odont/o (teeth)

Laryng/o (larynx)

Trache/o (trachea)

Bronchiol/o (bronchioles)

Pneum/o, Pneumon/o, Pulmon/o (lung)

Gastr/o (stomach)

Col/o or Colon/o (colon)

Enter/o (small intestine) three parts: duoden/o
                                         jejun/o
                                         ile/o

Salping/o (fallopian tube)

Sigmoid/o (part of colon)

Hyster/o or Metro (uterus)

Cervic/o (cervix) neck of uterus

Colp/o (vagina)

Figure 1 - Gyne (woman). Anterior view showing intestinal tract, female reproductive organs, lung and airway. Redrawn after Prendergast A (1983) Medical Terminology, 2nd edn. Addison-Wesley.

ROOTS FOR BODY PARTS AND ORGANS

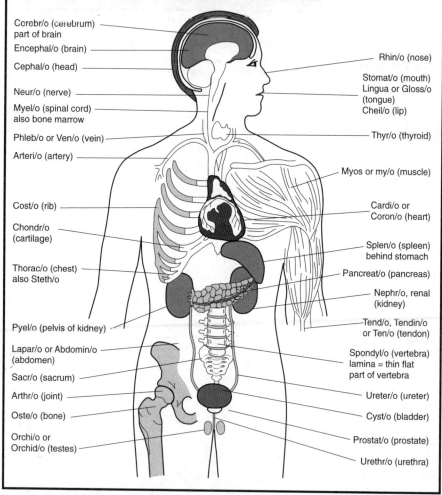

Cerebr/o (cerebrum) part of brain

Encephal/o (brain)

Cephal/o (head)

Neur/o (nerve)

Myel/o (spinal cord) also bone marrow

Phleb/o or Ven/o (vein)

Arteri/o (artery)

Cost/o (rib)

Chondr/o (cartilage)

Thorac/o (chest) also Steth/o

Pyel/o (pelvis of kidney)

Lapar/o or Abdomin/o (abdomen)

Sacr/o (sacrum)

Arthr/o (joint)

Oste/o (bone)

Orchi/o or Orchid/o (testes)

Rhin/o (nose)

Stomat/o (mouth)
Lingua or Gloss/o (tongue)
Cheil/o (lip)

Thyr/o (thyroid)

Myos or my/o (muscle)

Cardi/o or Coron/o (heart)

Splen/o (spleen) behind stomach

Pancreat/o (pancreas)

Nephr/o, renal (kidney)

Tend/o, Tendin/o or Ten/o (tendon)

Spondyl/o (vertebra) lamina = thin flat part of vertebra

Ureter/o (ureter)

Cyst/o (bladder)

Prostat/o (prostate)

Urethr/o (urethra)

Figure 2 - Andro (man). Anterior view showing male reproductive organs, urinary tract, heart, spleen, pancreas, hip joint and some shoulder muscles. Redrawn after Prendergast A (1983) Medical Terminology, 2nd edn. Addison-Wesley.

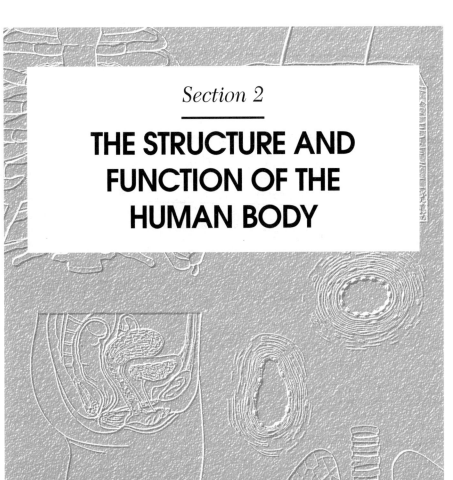

Section 2
___

THE STRUCTURE AND FUNCTION OF THE HUMAN BODY

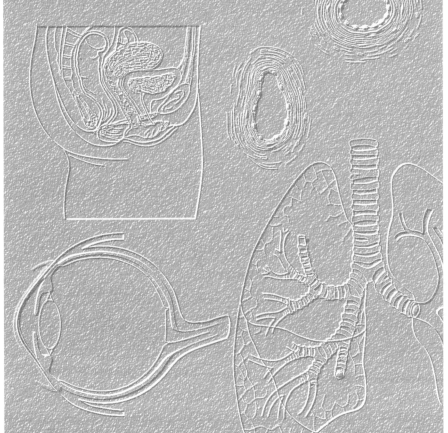

ANATOMY

Anatomy is the study of the structure of the body.

PHYSIOLOGY

Physiology is the study of the function of the body.

The basic elements

The human body is an incredibly complex creation, much of which is still not fully understood. In order to appreciate its complexity, the basic elements must be examined. The following are the main structures of which it is composed:

- Cells
- Tissues
- Organs
- Systems

Cells

The human body is composed of billions of tiny living materials known as cells. Cells vary in form and size, each type being adapted in structure to the function it performs.

The cell is composed of **protoplasm** containing numerous inclusions. It is surrounded by a selective semi-permeable membrane; i.e. it will allow some substances in and out through the membrane, but not others.

At some stage in every cell's life, there is a **nucleus** surrounded by a similar membrane known as the **nuclear membrane** (see Figure 3). It is here within the nucleus that the chromosomes are found, consisting of **DNA** (deoxyribonucleic acid). Each human cell normally contains 23 pairs of **chromosomes**, and it is upon these structures that the genetic blueprint is found, known as **genes**. These determine the individual characteristics of each cell.

The sex cells (**gametes**) of the ovum from the female and the spermatazoon from the male contain only 23 single chromosomes, which upon fusion at fertilisation enables the mixing of the genetic materials to form a new unique human being.

Tissues

Similar types of cells are grouped together to form tissues (see Figure 4). Each type of tissue has a particular function.

Abbreviations

Ca	carcinoma
SA	sarcoma
TNM	tumour nodes metastases
T	tumour

Types of tissues

There are four main types of tissue in the human body:

1. **Epithelial**   covering and lining of organs and cavities, (known as endothelium when lining internal organs).

2. **Connective**   supporting tissue, includes fibrous and elastic fibres, ligaments, cartilage and bone-blood.

3. **Muscle**   **voluntary muscle** (skeletal) attached to the skeleton; **involuntary muscle** (smooth)

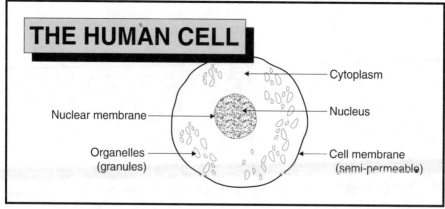

THE HUMAN CELL

Cytoplasm

Nuclear membrane

Nucleus

Organelles (granules)

Cell membrane (semi-permeable)

Figure 3 - The human cell.

TISSUE CELLS

A EPITHELIUM

(i) Simple squamous 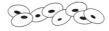 Line blood vessel (smooth)

(ii) Cuboid 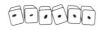 Produce secretions e.g. mucus

(iii) Columnar 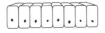 Line glands and digestive systems

(iv) Ciliated 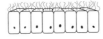 Line air passages and fallopian tube

(v) Stratified squamous 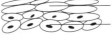 Horny stratified layer - no nucleus
Germinative layer of skin

(vi) Transitional 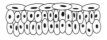 Found in bladder, capable of withstanding urine

B CONNECTIVE

(i) White fibrous (e.g. ligaments) Collagen fibres

(ii) Yellow elastic (e.g. elastic cartilage) White fibrous and yellow elastic

(iii) Areolar (e.g. subcutaneous tissue) 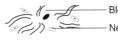 Blood vessel — Nerve fibre

Packing tissue Combination of white fibres yellow elastic and cells

(iv) Adipose (e.g. around the kidneys) 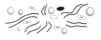 Similar to areolar, but containing many fat cells

Figure 4 - Tissue cells.

forming many internal organs, e.g. the stomach; **cardiac muscle** is a specialised muscle found only in the heart.

4. **Nerve**   a highly specialised tissue containing neurones forming the central, autonomic and peripheral nervous systems as well as special sensory organs, e.g. retina of eye (see Section 13).

Organs

Differing types of tissues are grouped together to form organs which perform special functions.

Systems

Organs working together to perform particular functions are known as systems. In health, each system normally works in harmony with others to maintain the body in its correct state (homeostasis).

PROPERTIES OF LIVING ORGANISMS

All living organisms, as opposed to non-living matter, have the following qualities:

Respiration   the process of producing energy in order to carry out all the metabolic processes required. In humans, this involves the absorption of oxygen for use in the cells together with glucose, and the production of waste products for excretion of carbon dioxide and water.

Nutrition   the process by which food is obtained for use as energy for growth or repair of the body.

Excretion   the process by which the body eliminates the waste products of metabolism.

Growth and repair   the ability to increase in size and repair damage to cells as well as producing new, similar cells (by **mitosis** division).

Reproduction   the process by which new individuals are produced (by **meiosis** division).

Sensitivity   the ability to detect changes in the environment.

Movement   capability of some movement.

NON-LIVING MATERIALS

The following materials are also present in the body and are essential to life:

Water - H_2O forming the largest component of all.

Mineral salts including:

Sodium	Na
Potassium	K
Calcium	Ca
Magnesium	Mg
Iron	Fe

Phosphates, carbonates, chlorides and other trace elements.

The balance of salts in the body is vital to life, and the electrolytes or electrolytic balance (balance of ions or mineral salts) are often measured in blood tests.

METABOLISM

Metabolism is the basic working of the body cells. It concerns the continuous chemical changes which occur to sustain life. Energy is produced as a by-product of the reactions.

OSMOSIS

This is the passage of fluid across a semi-permeable membrane, which allows equalisation of the concentration of solutions either side of the membrane. Tissue fluid is drawn back into the venous capillaries of the body by the presence of large plasma proteins, after it has given up its nutrients etc. to the tissue cells.

GLANDS

These are structures which produce and secrete their own substance. There are two types:

1. **Exocrine glands (with ducts)**
   These pour their secretions through ducts to another organ, or directly upon the surface of a membrane, e.g. mucus secretions from epithelial tissue, or **bile** from the liver to the bile-duct.

2. **Endocrine glands (ductless)**

2. Endocrine glands (ductless)

These produce secretions known as **hormones**, which are secreted directly into the blood supply for stimulation of another target organ (see Section 15, Endocrine system).

MEMBRANES

These are special tissues covering and lining areas of the body. They consist of:

Mucous membranes	tissue containing mucus-secreting cells which moisten and lubricate surfaces.
Serous membranes	a double-layered tissue composed of smooth, simple squamous epithelial cells which secrete a thin fluid between the two layers known as serous fluid, e.g. **pleura** covering the lungs and **peritoneum** covering abdominal organs.
Synovial membranes	a single membrane which produces a thick glairy fluid known as synovial fluid, found at freely moveable joints preventing friction and wear.

ANATOMICAL POSITION

The body is described facing forwards, feet apart,

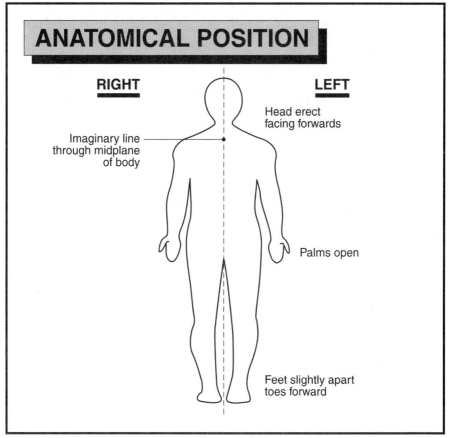

ANATOMICAL POSITION

RIGHT   **LEFT**

Imaginary line through midplane of body

Head erect facing forwards

Palms open

Feet slightly apart toes forward

Figure 5 - Anatomical position.

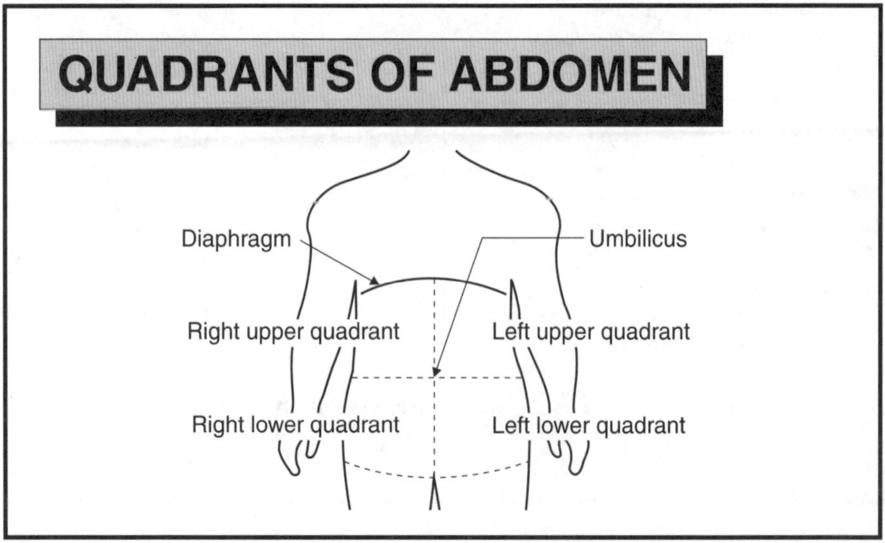

QUADRANTS OF ABDOMEN

Figure 6 - Quadrants of abdominopelvic regions of the body.

arms at sides and palms facing forward, as illustrated in Figure 5.

CAVITIES OF THE BODY

The main cavities of the body are the:

- **Thoracic cavity**
- **Abdominal cavity**
- **Pelvic cavity**

REGIONS OF THE ABDOMEN

The abdominal and pelvic areas of the trunk are divided into **quadrants**, as shown in Figure 6. The abdomen is also divided into the regions shown in Figure 7 (opposite).

TERMINOLOGY

Atrophy	wastage of an organ
Cytology	study of cells.
Histology	study of tissues.
Hypertropy	enlargement of an organ with its own tissue
Infarct	a wedge-shaped area of tissue deprived of its blood supply
Ischaemia	lack of blood to a part
Oncology	study of tumours.

DISEASES AND DISORDERS

Adenoma	tumour of a gland.
Benign	favourable for recovery, opposite of malignant.
Carcinoma	cancerous, abnormal malignant cells growing in the body.
Chondroma	benign tumour of cartilage.
Chondrosarcoma	malignant tumour of cartilage and bone.
Contusion	bleeding beneath the skin (bruise).
Embolism	obstruction of a blood vessel by a detached, travelling particle of blood, fat or air.
Embolus	blood clot, fat or air detached from another place and travelling in the blood stream.
Epithelioma	tumour of epithelial tissue (lining and covering organs), e.g. of the epidermis.
Fibroma	tumour of fibrous tissue.
Fibrosis	formation of scar tissue.
Haematoma	swelling containing blood.
Hilum	a depression on the surface of an organ where blood and other

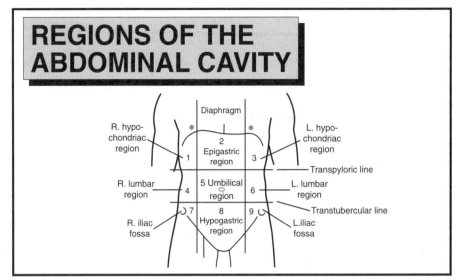

REGIONS OF THE ABDOMINAL CAVITY

Diaphragm

R. hypo-chondriac region

2 Epigastric region

L. hypo-chondriac region

Transpyloric line

1

3

R. lumbar region

4

5 Umbilical region

6

L. lumbar region

Transtubercular line

7

8 Hypogastric region

9

R. iliac fossa

L.iliac fossa

Figure 7 - Regions of the abdominal cavity.

vessels, and ducts enter and leave.

Ischaemia	deficiency of blood supply to a part.
Keloid scar	abnormal overgrowth of fibrous tissue in the healing of a wound.
Lesion	morbid (abnormal) change in tissue.
Lipoma	tumour composed of fat.
Malignant	virulent/dangerous, likely to have a fatal outcome (disease or tumour).
Myalgia	painful muscles.
Myasthenia gravis	disease causing abnormal fatigue and weakness in voluntary muscles.
Myoma	tumour composed of muscle.
NG	new growth.
Necrosis	death of tissue.
Necrotising fasciitis	destruction of soft tissue by overwhelming infection, usually post-operatively, by haemolytic streptococcus bacteria (Group A)
Neoplasm	new growth or tumour.
Oedema	free fluid in the tissues.
Papilloma	wart-type benign tumour.
Peritonitis	inflammation of the peritoneum (the lining of the abdomen and pelvic cavities).
Pleurisy	inflammation of the pleura (the covering of the lungs).
Sarcoma	cancer arising in the connective tissue, e.g. bone, blood.
Sebaceous cyst	swelling caused by blockage of sebaceous gland duct in the skin.

PROCEDURES AND EQUIPMENT

Biopsy	removal of a portion of living tissue for micro-scopic investigation.

CLASSIFICATION OF DISEASES

Congenital	present at birth
Acquired	acquired after birth
Acute	rapid onset and progress
Allergic	hypersensitivity to for-eign proteins
Chronic	slow onset and

Chronic	slow onset and progress	
Cryptogenic	of doubtful or hidden origin	
Endocrine	associated with hormone dysfunction	
Familial	occurs in families	
Functional	no anatomical abnormality demonstrated but associated with dysfunction	
Iatrogenic	a disease produced by the treatment given for a primary illness	
Idiopathic	peculiar to the individual	
Infectious	caused by microorganisms readily passed on to other people	
Metabolic	disorder of basic working (physiology) of the body	
Neoplastic	associated with development of new growths (e.g. malignant or benign tumours)	
Organic	structural abnormality demonstrated	
Silent	no symptoms apparent or obvious signs	
Systemic	involving the entire body	
Traumatic	involving injury	
Local	involving an area or one part of the body only	

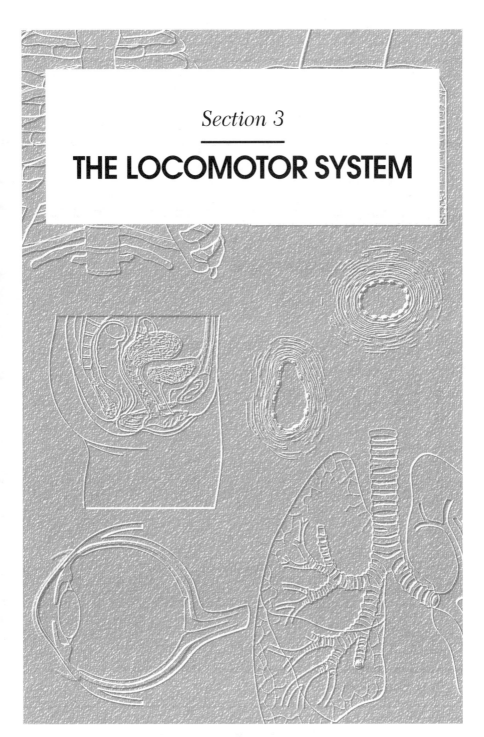

Section 3

THE LOCOMOTOR SYSTEM

This consists of the bones, muscles, ligaments, cartilage and tendons, and is mainly concerned with movement.

BONE

There are two different types of bone structure known as:

- **Compact** (hard)
- **Cancellous** (spongy)

Cancellous bone tissue forms the red bone marrow. All bones are covered in a membrane known as the **periosteum**, which provides nourishment.

Hyaline cartilage tissue is found at the ends of long bones where joints are formed, preventing wear. In fetal life, bone is generally developed from cartilage tissue by the laying down of calcium salts by specialised bone cells. This continues after birth and is known as **ossification**. **Vitamin D** and **calcium** are essential for healthy bone formation. There are 206 bones in the adult human body.

SKELETON

This is made up of five classifications of bones:

1. **long bones**   forming limbs and having a cavity.

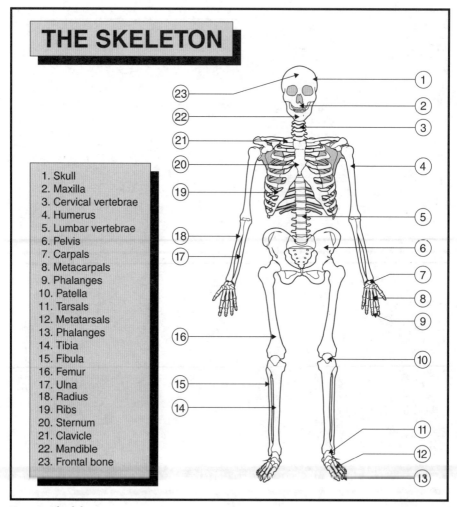

THE SKELETON

1. Skull
2. Maxilla
3. Cervical vertebrae
4. Humerus
5. Lumbar vertebrae
6. Pelvis
7. Carpals
8. Metacarpals
9. Phalanges
10. Patella
11. Tarsals
12. Metatarsals
13. Phalanges
14. Tibia
15. Fibula
16. Femur
17. Ulna
18. Radius
19. Ribs
20. Sternum
21. Clavicle
22. Mandible
23. Frontal bone

Figure 8 - The skeleton.

THE SKULL BONES

1. Parietal*
2. Sphenoid*
3. Temporal*
4. Occipital*
5. Mastoid portion
   of temporal lobe
6. Mandible
7. Malar or zygomatic
8. Maxilla
9. Ethmoid*
10. Nasal
11. Lacrimal
12. Frontal*
   *Form the cranium

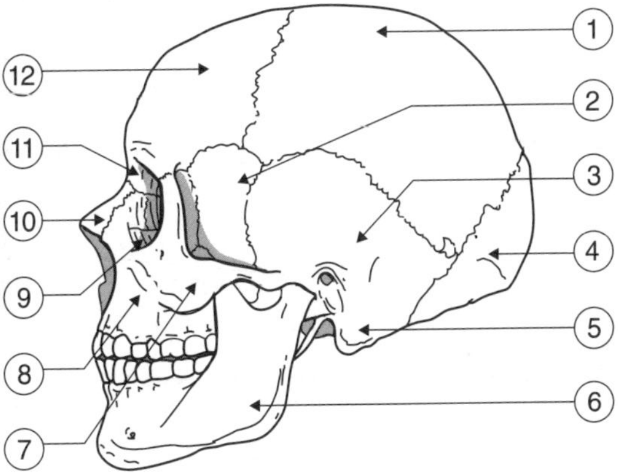

Figure 9 - Bones of the skull.

2. **short bones** — having no cavity, found in the hands and feet.

3. **flat bones** — forming the cranium and scapula.

4. **irregular bones** — face bones and vertebrae.

5. **sesamoid bones** — formed in a tendon, e.g. patella and hyoid bones.

The bony framework of the body (see Figure 8) has the following functions:

Support — provides a framework for the body and gives shape.

Leverage — provides levers for muscle attachment allowing movement and articulation.

Protection — protects organs, e.g. brain within the cranium.

Storage — stores calcium salts.

Production — manufactures blood cells in the bone marrow.

There are two parts to the skeleton:

1. The **axial skeleton** - formed from the skull, vertebrae, rib cage and breast bone - made up of 80 bones.
2. The **appendicular skeleton** - consisting of 126 bones forming the limb bones and their girdles.

THE SKULL

This includes the bones of the face and the bones which form the **cranium** containing the brain and beginning of the spinal cord (see Figure 9). The lobes of the **cerebrum** (part of brain) are named by the bones under which they lie.

Bones of the cranium

These consist of the following individual bones:

- One **occipital**
- Two **parietal**
- Two **temporal**
- One **frontal**
- One **sphenoid**
- One **ethmoid**

Fontanelles

The uniting of the cranial bones by **sutures** (fibrous immovable joints) occurs after birth. Because the bones are not united in the fetus, moulding of the skull to aid delivery is able to occur during childbirth.

The anterior fontanelle is a 'soft spot' which can be felt until its closure at approximately 18 months. The 'soft spot' allows the skull bones to continue to grow to accommodate the increasing size of the brain.

The posterior fontanelle closes at approximately three months (see Figure 10).

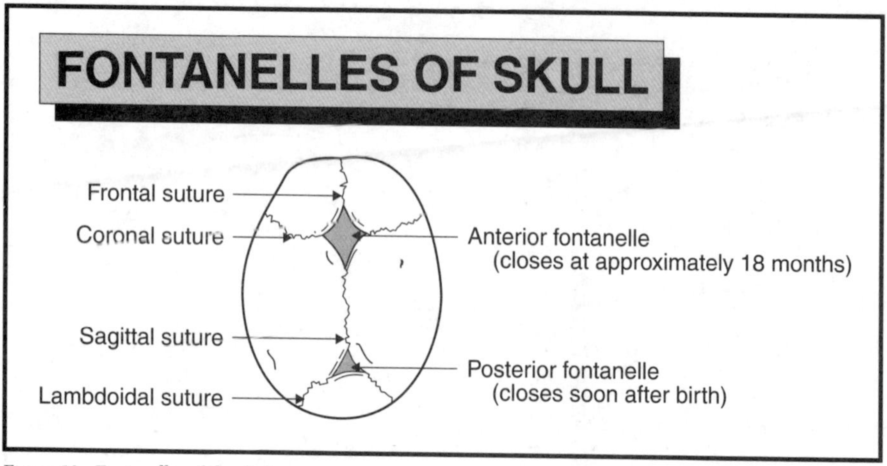

FONTANELLES OF SKULL

Frontal suture —

Coronal suture —

Anterior fontanelle
(closes at approximately 18 months)

Sagittal suture —

Lambdoidal suture —

Posterior fontanelle
(closes soon after birth)

Figure 10 - Fontanelles of the skull.

Bones of the face

These consist of the following individual bones:

- One **mandible** - lower jaw
- Two **maxilla** - upper jaw
- Two **malar** or **zygomatic** - cheek bones
- One **nasal** - part of nose
- One **vomer** - part of nasal septum
- Two **lacrimal** (lacrymal) - bony orbit
- Two **palatine** - hard palate in mouth
- Two **turbinate** - inside nose

Air sinuses of the skull

These are cavities containing air within the bone tissues which lighten the skull. They are lined with mucous membrane which may become infected. They are found in the following bones:

- **Frontal**
- **Maxillary**
- **Ethmoid**
- **Sphenoid**

Hyoid bone

The **hyoid** bone is a small bone to which the tongue is attached. It is often found to be fractured in cases of strangulation.

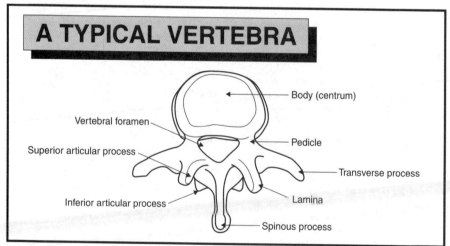

A TYPICAL VERTEBRA

Body (centrum)

Vertebral foramen

Pedicle

Superior articular process

Transverse process

Inferior articular process

Lamina

Spinous process

Figure 11 - A typical vertebra.

VERTEBRAE

There are 33 irregular bones in the vertebral column or **spine**, stacked one upon the other and bound together by strong ligaments. The spine combines great strength with mobility. Its function is to:

- Provide a framework for attachment of other structures.
- Protect the spinal cord and nerves.
- Provide locomotion.
- Absorb shock.
- Form strong joints.

Vertebrae are in groups and are named after the region in which they are situated. They become larger and heavier in size as they descend, although the neural or vertebral **foramen** (hole through which the spinal cord travels) becomes smaller.

The vertebrae are described as **typical** (having similar features) or **atypical** (not having the typical features).

Typical vertebrae

A typical vertebra (see Figure 11) contains the following features:

- A **body**.
- Four **articulating processes** (surfaces) - forming joints with the vertebrae above and below.
- Two **pedicles**.
- Two **transverse processes**.
- Two **lamina**.
- A **spinous process** - formed from the uniting of the lamina.
- Two **intervertebral notches** - through which spinal nerves travel from each side of the spinal cord.
- A **vertebral (neural) foramen** - through which the spinal cord travels.

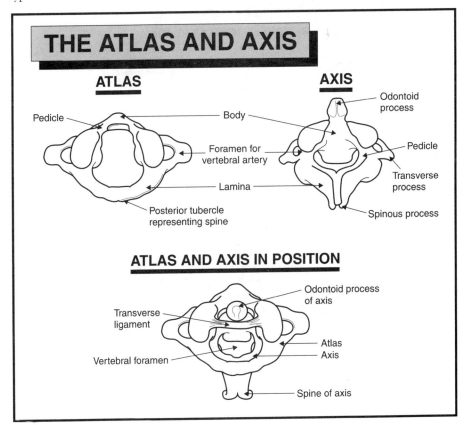

THE ATLAS AND AXIS

ATLAS

Pedicle

Body

Foramen for vertebral artery

Lamina

Posterior tubercle representing spine

AXIS

Odontoid process

Pedicle

Transverse process

Spinous process

ATLAS AND AXIS IN POSITION

Transverse ligament

Vertebral foramen

Odontoid process of axis

Atlas

Axis

Spine of axis

Figure 12 - The atlas and axis (anterior view).

Atypical vertebrae

These consist of the **atlas** and **axis** (the first and second cervical vertebrae), and the **sacrum** and **coccyx** which are formed of fused vertebrae. They do **not** possess the typical features described above.

The atlas forms a joint (**articulates**) with the occipital bone of the skull above, and allows the movement of nodding the head. The atlas and axis form a pivot joint which allows movement of the head from side to side (see Figure 12).

Intervertebral discs

Between the bodies of each vertebra are the intervertebral discs, pads of cartilage filled with a fluid. These act as shock absorbers, preventing damage to the structure.

Regions of the vertebral column

- **cervical**   seven bones
- **thoracic**   12 bones
- **lumbar**   five bones
- **sacral**   five fused bones
- **coccyx**   four fused bones

Curvatures

The curvatures of the vertebral column are initially formed in fetal development, while the developing fetus is curled up in the mother's uterus. These are

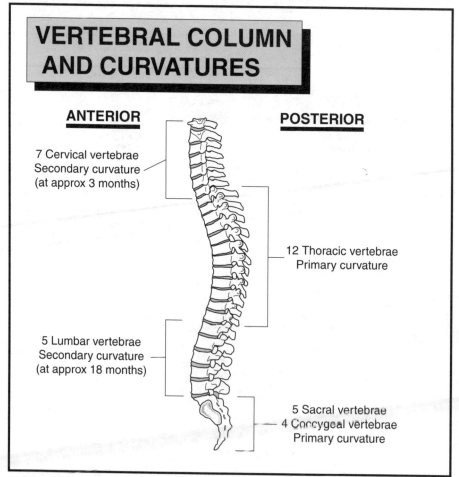

VERTEBRAL COLUMN AND CURVATURES

ANTERIOR

7 Cervical vertebrae
Secondary curvature
(at approx 3 months)

5 Lumbar vertebrae
Secondary curvature
(at approx 18 months)

POSTERIOR

12 Thoracic vertebrae
Primary curvature

5 Sacral vertebrae
4 Coccygeal vertebrae
Primary curvature

Figure 13 - The vertebral column and curvatures.

the **thoracic** and **sacral** curvatures (see Figure 13).

After birth, the **cervical curvature** is formed when the baby is able to support its own head, from approximately three months. The **lumbar curvature** forms when the child stands and supports his/her body at 12-18 months.

RIB CAGE (THORACIC)

This is made up of the following structures (see Figure 14):

- One **sternum (breast bone)**
- Twelve pairs of **ribs**
- Twelve **thoracic vertebrae**

Sternum

This flat bone forms the front (**anterior**) part of the rib cage, and it is to this that the ribs and collar bone (**clavicle**) are attached. It is composed of three parts known as the **manubrium, body** and **xiphoid** portions. Beneath this bone lies the heart, and it is this bone which is depressed in the rendering of **cardiopulmonary resuscitation (CPR)**.

The ribs form the bony lateral walls of the chest cavity and form joints (**articulate**) with the **thoracic vertebrae** at the rear (**posteriorly**). The first 10 pairs of ribs are attached to the sternum **anteriorly** by the attachment of **costal cartilages**, the first seven directly and the lower three indirectly as shown in Figure 14. The last two pairs of ribs are known as **floating ribs** as they remain unattached to the sternum.

The rib cage protects the organs lying within it: heart, lungs, oesophagus, major blood vessels etc.

Intercostal muscles are attached to the ribs between the rib spaces and are involved in the process of **inspiration** and **expiration**. The rib cage swings outwards and upwards on inspiration, which increases the capacity of the thoracic cavity, allowing expansion of the lung tissue (see Section 7).

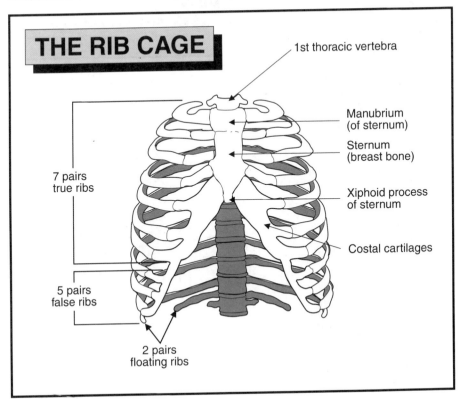

THE RIB CAGE

1st thoracic vertebra

Manubrium (of sternum)

Sternum (breast bone)

Xiphoid process of sternum

Costal cartilages

7 pairs true ribs

5 pairs false ribs

2 pairs floating ribs

Figure 14 - The rib cage.

PELVIS

This structure is composed of the following bones:

- Two **innominate bones**
- **Sacrum** (part of the vertebrae)

These structures are bound together by ligaments to form the pelvic basin (see Figure 15). The innominate bone is composed of three separate bones which are fused together:

- Ilium
- Ischium
- Pubis

The area within the pelvis is known as the **pelvic cavity** and contains important structures, such as the intestine, rectum and anus, bladder, ureters, urethra, prostate gland, some organs of the male reproductive system, female reproductive organs, blood vessels, nerves etc., which are protected by the bony frame.

JOINTS

These are formed wherever two or more bony surfaces are attached to each other.

Types of joint (see Figure 16)

- **fixed joints** — formed of fibrous tissue where no movement is possible, e.g. sutures of cranium.

- **slightly moveable** — cartilaginous joints which allow only slight movement, e.g. intervertebral joints between the bodies of vertebrae.

- **freely moveable** — synovial joints which allow free movement according to the shape of the joint.

Synovial joints are lined with a synovial membrane which produces synovial fluid, a thick glairy fluid which acts as a lubricant preventing friction and wear. The ends of the bones which form these joints are covered in **hyaline cartilage** (see Figure 17).

BURSA

This is a sac lined with synovial membrane containing synovial fluid, usually found between a

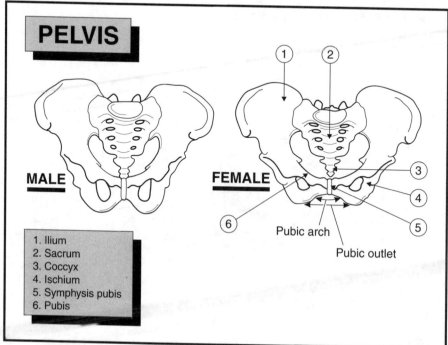

PELVIS

MALE

FEMALE

1 2

3

4

6

5

Pubic arch

Pubic outlet

1. Ilium
2. Sacrum
3. Coccyx
4. Ischium
5. Symphysis pubis
6. Pubis

Figure 15 - The pelvis.

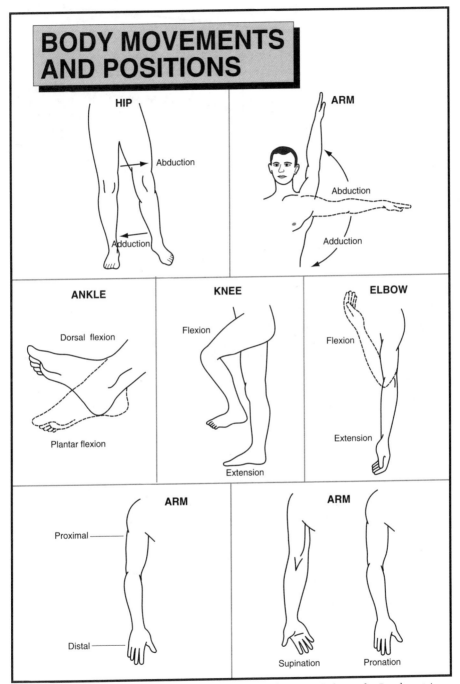

Figure 16 - A sample of terms used to describe body movements and positions. Redrawn after Prendergast A (1983) Medical Terminology, 2nd edn. Addison-Wesley.

tendon and a bone near the surface of the body in order to prevent friction on movement. Inflammation of these is common in conditions such as **housemaid's knee**.

LIGAMENTS

These are composed of tough fibrous tissue and bind bone to bone.

MUSCLES

These are strong elastic tissue, well supplied with blood (vascular), capable of contraction and relaxation. In life, muscles are always partially contracted, and this is known as muscle tone.

Types of muscle

There are three types of muscle in the body:

1. **Voluntary** (striated) attached to the skeleton and under control of the will.

2. **Involuntary** (unstriated) smooth and controlled automatically by the autonomic nervous system; these form the walls of major organs, e.g. stomach.

3. **Cardiac** (myogenic) special muscle exclusive to the heart, forming its walls; controlled by the autonomic nervous system. It's capable of independent contraction causing quivering of the heart if the nerve supply within is interrupted.

Skeletal or striated muscle is often named from its shape, e.g. **deltoid** (triangular), or the number of heads it has, e.g. **triceps**. Muscles usually work in groups and in co-ordination.

DIAPHRAGM

This is an important muscle which divides the **thoracic** (chest) cavity from the abdominal cavity. It is essential for the act of respiration (breathing). Also involved are the **intercostal muscles** which move the rib cage (see Section 7).

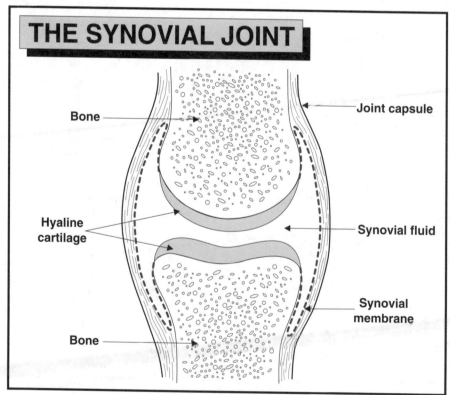

THE SYNOVIAL JOINT

Bone

Joint capsule

Hyaline cartilage

Synovial fluid

Synovial membrane

Bone

Figure 17 - A synovial joint.

TENDONS

These are specialised fibrous bands found at the ends of muscles which attach muscle to bone, or muscle to muscle.

ENERGY

Muscles require a good blood supply to provide oxygen and nutrients. Glucose is converted and stored in muscle tissue ready for its release when required. Cramp occurs when there is insufficient oxygen available for the chemical reaction to occur and **lactic acid** is produced. The remedy for cramp is to extend the muscle.

HERNIA

This condition arises from a weakness in the muscle which allows part of an organ to **prolapse** through the space created by the weakness.

Types of hernia

Inguinal hernia

This is common in men. It arises in an area known as the **inguinal canal**, which is a tunnel in the abdominal muscles where the spermatic cord and testis travel to descend into the scrotum in fetal life. Protrusion of the intestine through this area can occur and may lead to **strangulation**, i.e. the blood supply to this intestinal area becomes deprived.

Femoral hernia

This is a condition where the weakness is in the groin where the **femoral artery** travels to the leg. Hernias in this area are more common among women.

Hiatus hernia

This is a condition where the weakness is in the diaphragm. Part of the **oesophagus** (gullet) and/or the stomach travels through the space created by the weakness causing symptoms of 'heart burn' due to gastric juices affecting the oesophagus.

Umbilical hernia

In this condition, the weakness is in the area of muscle through which the **umbilical cord** travelled in the fetus and may give rise to an intestinal protrusion.

ABBREVIATIONS

BI	bone injury
C1, C2 etc	cervical vertebrae
CDH	congenital dislocation of the hip
CPT	carpal tunnel syndrome
L1, L2 etc	lumbar vertebrae
NBI	no bone injury
OA	osteoarthritis
PID	prolapsed intervertebral disc (can also mean pelvic inflammatory disease)
RA	rheumatoid arthritis
RTA	road traffic accident
T1, T2 etc	thoracic vertebrae
THR	total hip relacement
TKR	total knee replacement

TERMINOLOGY

Arthr/o	stem for joint.
Articul/o	joint.
Chondr/o	stem for cartilage.
Cost/o	stem for rib.
Crani/o	stem for cranium (skull containing brain).
Ili/o	stem for ilium (bone of pelvis).
My/o (myos)	stem for muscle.
Myel/o	stem for bone marrow (also spinal cord).
Oste/o	stem for bone.
Spondyl/o (vertebr/o)	stem for vertebra.
Synov/o	synovial.
Ten/o, tendin/o	tendon.

DISEASES AND DISORDERS

Ankylosing spondylitis	fixation of the vertebrae with fibrous tissue causing loss of movement.
Ankylosis	immobilisation and solidification of a joint.
Arthritis	inflammation of a joint.
Arthrodynia	pain in a joint.
Bursitis	inflammation of the pad of synovial membrane protecting a bone near the surface of the body, e.g. the elbow or knee
Callus	an outgrowth of partly bony tissue produced in the body's process of the mending of bones.

Exostosis	an overgrowth of bone.
Genu valgum	knock knee.
Genu varum	bow legged.
Hallux valgus	bunion/deviation of the large toe joint.
Kyphosis	hunchback/excessive curvature of the thoracic vertebrae.
Lordosis	'sway back'/excessive inward curvature of the lumbar spine.
Luxation	complete dislocation of a joint
Osteoarthritis	degenerative disease of ageing - large joints of knee, hip etc.
Osteoma	tumour of bone.
Osteomalacia	rickets - softening of bone due to lack of vitamin D and deposit of calcium salts.
Osteomyelitis	inflammation of the bone marrow.
Osteoporosis	brittle bones due to ageing and lack of oestrogen hormone which affects the ability to deposit calcium in the matrix of bone.
Polyarthritis	arthritis involving many joints.
Rheumatoid arthritis	disease causing inflammation of small joints, usually hands and feet.
Scoliosis	a lateral S-shaped deformity of the vertebrae.
Spina bifida	failure of the spinous processes to unite in fetal development, causing various degrees of deformity, with or without the meninges (covering of spinal cord) and/or spinal cord protruding through to the surface of the body.
Spondylitis	inflammation of one or more vertebrae.
Spondylosis	degenerative disease of the spine, crumbling occurs.
Still's disease	a form of rheumatoid polyarthritis in children.

Subluxation	partial dislocation of a joint.
Synovitis	inflammation of a synovial (moveable) joint.
Talipes	club foot deformity.
Valgus	deviation outwards.
Varus	deviation inwards.

PROCEDURES AND EQUIPMENT

Arthroclasia	surgical breaking of a joint to provide movement.
Arthrocentesis	puncture of a joint cavity to remove fluid.
Arthrodesis	surgical stiffening of a joint.
Arthroplasty	reshaping or moulding of a joint.
Arthroscopy	examination of a joint with a lighted instrument.
Bursectomy	removal (excision) of bursa.
Laminectomy	surgical removal of the lamina of a vertebra to relieve pressure in 'slipped disc.'
Meniscectomy	surgical removal of the semi-lunar cartilage of the knee joint.
Open reduction	using surgery to reduce a dislocation of a joint or fracture as oppposed to a closed reduction where manipulation alone is used.
Osteotomy	cutting or dividing of bone.
Prosthesis	artificial part or replacement, e.g. hip, leg or breast.
Synovectomy	surgical removal of synovial (lining) membrane.
Tenotomy	surgical dividing or cutting of a tendon.

FRACTURES

Fracture	a break in the continuity of the bone - includes cracks as well as complete breaks. (See Figure 18 for types of fracture.)

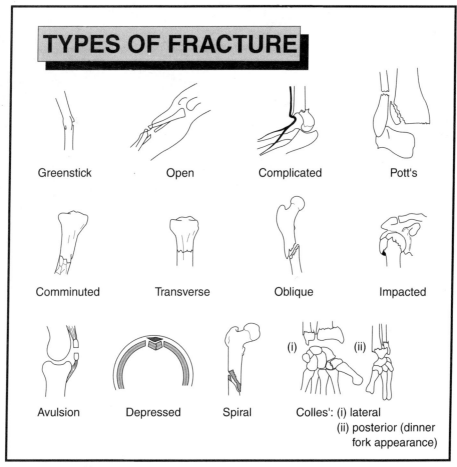

TYPES OF FRACTURE

Greenstick · Open · Complicated · Pott's

Comminuted · Transverse · Oblique · Impacted

Avulsion · Depressed · Spiral · Colles': (i) lateral (ii) posterior (dinner fork appearance)

Figure 18 - Types of fracture.

Avulsion	fragmented bone at the site of a ligament or tendon attachment.
Colles'	fracture of the wrist, both the radius and ulna are fractured and cause the typical dinner fork deformity.
Comminuted	a fracture where there are several breaks in the bone.
Complicated	fracture in which there is associated damage to vital neighbouring structures.
Compound/open	a break in a bone where there is communication with the outside air through the skin - danger of infection.
Depressed	fracture of the skull with depressed segments.
Greenstick	type of fracture in children where the bone does not completely break as it is not as ossified (hardened with mineral salts), but is rather like a green branch of a tree in its splitting - heals quickly.

| **Impacted** | a fracture where the ends of the bone are forced into one another. | **Pott's** | fracture of the ankle involving both the tibia and fibula. |
| **Oblique** | fracture that is not directly across the axis of the bone. | **Transverse** | fracture at right angles to the axis of the bone. |

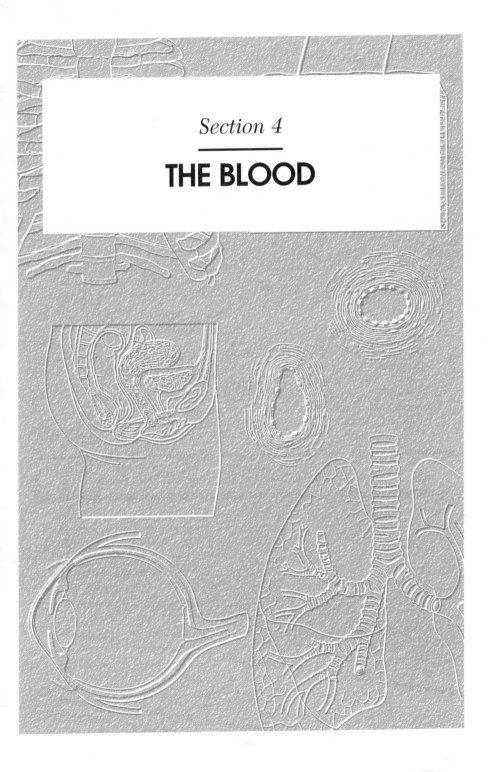

Section 4

THE BLOOD

FUNCTION

This can be summarised as both the transportation of substances throughout the body and also a defence system.

STRUCTURE

Blood consists of a slightly alkaline (pH 7.35) straw-coloured fluid known as plasma that contains blood cells suspended within it. It is the main transport system of the body, travelling within a closed system of blood vessels.

An adult has eight to 10 pints (five to six litres) of blood.

PLASMA

The fluid which forms 55% of the blood and contains numerous substances, including:

- **Water** - 91%.
- **Mineral salts** - including sodium chloride, the largest component at 0.9%.
- **Food materials**
  - amino acids (proteins)
  - glucose
  - fats known as lipids.
- **Plasma proteins** - albumin, globulin and the clotting factors fibrinogen and prothrombin.
- **Waste materials** - carbon dioxide in solution, urea and uric acid.

- **Antibodies and antitoxins**
- **Vitamins**
- **Hormones**
- **Enzymes**
- **Oxygen** - in solution.

SERUM

When the clotting factor fibrinogen has been removed from plasma, it is known as serum.

CELLS

These consist of three main groups (see Figure 19):

- **Red cells** known as **erythrocytes** (around 5 million per cubic millimetre – see Tables 1 and 2).
- **White cells** known as **leucocytes** (around 8,000 per cubic millimetre).
- **Platelets** known as **thrombocytes** (around 350,000 per cubic millimetre).

Erythrocytes

These are smaller than the white cells and have no nuclei. This gives them a biconcave shape and enables them to carry more **haemoglobin** (an orange-coloured substance containing iron, which combines with oxygen in the blood contained in the capillary network of the lungs). This is then carried in the blood stream, ready to supply the tissues where oxygen is released. Their function is to carry oxygen, and they are

Table I – Meanings of pathology values for red blood cells

Term	Meaning of term
Erythrocyte count	number of red blood cells per litre or per cubic millimetre of blood
Haemoglobin	weight of haemoglobin in whole blood expressed as grams per decilitre
Mean cell volume	average volume of cells expressed in femtolitres
Mean corpuscular (cell) haemoglobin	average amount of haemoglobin in each cell expressed in femtolitres
Mean corpuscular (cell) haemoglobin concentration	amount of haemoglobin in 100 ml (1 decilitre) of blood
Packed cell volume or haemocrit	volume of red cells in 1 litre (100 millilitres) of whole blood

small enough to travel within the capillaries. Haemoglobin combines with oxygen to form oxyhaemoglobin:

$$\text{Haemoglobin} + O_2 \leftrightarrow \text{oxyhaemoglobin}$$
(reversible)

Erythrocytes are manufactured in the bone marrow, live for approximately 3 months and are destroyed by the spleen and liver. The part containing iron is stored by the liver and the residue is excreted as bile pigments (bilirubin) in the faeces, and it is this pigment which gives the faeces their colour.

ANAEMIA

Anaemia may be defined as a condition in which there is an insufficient amount of oxygen-carrying capacity in the blood. It may be caused by too few normal erythrocytes or by red blood cells not being mature and fully charged with haemoglobin. Varying conditions of anaemia may give rise to erythrocytes which are large and pale (**macrocytic**) or small (**microcytic**).

Certain factors are necessary for the production of mature red blood cells. These include iron and trace elements as well as vitamin C and folic acid. **Vitamin B₁₂** is also essential and is known as the **extrinsic factor**. These are all provided in the diet.

Pernicious anaemia

However, a further substance known as **Castle's intrinsic factor**, found within the gastric juice produced by the stomach, is essential for the absorption of vitamin B_{12} necessary in the diet. If this is not present, a condition known as **pernicious anaemia** will result where large pale immature red cells (macrocytic), unable to carry much oxygen, occur. Treatment is by giving regular B_{12} injections.

Iron deficiency anameia

Iron deficiency anaemia is very common and occurs when there is insufficient iron or other necessary factors in the diet, or when there has been a loss of blood through haemorrhaging (bleeding), either severe or as a constant, slight loss, e.g. a slowly bleeding peptic ulcer. The condition of **menorrhagia** (heavy periods) is a common cause of this type of anaemia in women. The erythrocytes are pale (hypochromic) and small (microcytic).

Leucocytes

These white cells are composed of two main types:

    1. **Granulocytes (polymorphonuclear leucocytes)**; 65-75% of white cells.

Table 2 – Normal values of erythrocytes

Abbreviation	Sex	Normal value (For a meaning of these values see Section 17)
Erythrocyte count (RBC →red blood cells)	Female	$4.0-5.5 \times 10^{12}/l$ 4.0–5.5 million/mm³
	Male	$4.5-6.5 \times 10^{12}/l$ 4.5–6.5 million/mm³
Haemoglobin (Hb)	Female Male	11.5–16.5 g/dl 13.5–18.0 g/dl
Mean cell volume (MCV)		80–100 fl
Mean corpuscular (cell) haemoglobin concentration (MCHC)		30–36 g/dl of cells
Packed cell volume (PCV)	Female	0.37–0.47 l/l 37–47/mm³
Haematocrit (HCT)	Male	0.40–0.54 l/l 40–54/mm³

NB. There are variations of normal values with different laboratories

2. Non-granular leucocytes (mononuclear leucocytes); 25-35% of white cells.

The life-span of white cells is approximately 3 weeks or less and is dependent on the state of infection in the body.

Granulocytes (polymorphonuclear leucocytes)

These cells are manufactured in the bone marrow and are concerned with the defence of the body. They are mainly **phagocytes**, i.e. capable of changing their shape and ingesting (eating) bacteria and foreign matter. They are larger than the red cells but by changing their shape (**amoeboid action**) are able to squeeze out of the capillary walls to reach the tissues. Named after the stains which they will take up in the laboratory, they consist of three types:

- **Neutrophils** (60-70% of white cells)
- **Basophils** (0.5-2% of white blood cells)
- **Eosinophils** (2-4% of white blood cells)

The majority of this type of blood cell are neutrophils, which greatly increase in response to bacterial infection.

Non-granular (mononuclear) leucocytes

These blood cells consist of lymphocytes (representing 20-30% of blood cells) and monocytes (accounting for 4-8% of blood cells) and are developed in the bone marrow and lymph tissue.

Lymphocytes

These blood cells are concerned with immunity and when activated produce antibodies, so protecting the body from foreign materials e.g. viruses. These antibodies assist the other body

---

BLOOD CELLS

Average number per cubic millimetre of blood

RED CELLS (Erythrocytes)   5,000,000

Bioconcave discs
(contain no nucleus)

WHITE CELLS (Leucocytes)   8,000

Polymorphonuclear leucocytes
(or granulocytes)

Monocytes (mononuclear leucocytes
or non-granular leucocytes

Lymphocytes
(large or small)

PLATELETS OR THROMBOCYTES   350,000

Fragmented cells

Figure 19 - Blood cells.

34

defences to overcome infection. Lymphocytes form the majority of the non-granulocytes and are found in lymph tissue throughout the body.

Monocytes

These blood cells are also concerned with immunity and are capable of phagocytic and amoeboid action. They work in close association with lymphocytes and their numbers are greatly increased in certain infective conditions, e.g. glandular fever.

Thrombocytes

These are fragmented cells, with no nucleus, and are concerned with clotting. They are also manufactured in the bone marrow.

CLOTTING

The process of blood clotting requires many factors including thrombocytes (platelets). The clotting factors prothrombin, fibrinogen (manufactured in the liver) and vitamin K are essential.

Also necessary is factor VIII, a substance which is absent from the blood of patients suffering from haemophilia. This substance is given artificially by injection when necessary. Spontaneous bleeding occurs into joints with this condition.

BLOOD GROUPS

These are genetically determined. There are many different groups. The main classification is the Landsteiner ABO type (agglutinin) present in the red cells.

- **Type A** contains factor A in cells, anti-B in serum.
- **Type B** contains factor B in cells, anti-A in serum.
- **Type AB** contains factor A and B in cells, no anti-A or anti-B in serum.
- **Type O** contains no factor in cells anti-A and anti-B in serum.

Therefore the serum of group A blood, containing anti-B, will cause group B red blood cells to be destroyed and *vice versa*. The serum of group O blood will destroy A, B and AB. However, group AB blood will not react with any of the groups as it has no anti-factors in its serum to do so.

The Rhesus factor

A further factor present in the plasma of the blood is the Rhesus factor (anti-D) present in 85% of the population. When present the type is known as **Rhesus positive** (Rh +ve). When absent it is known as **Rhesus negative** (Rh -ve).

The Rhesus factor must always be considered, particularly in the case of females, where the giving of Rhesus-positive blood to someone who is Rhesus negative, will cause antibodies (anti-factors) to be produced by the person's immune system. Subsequently, in pregnancy, these can damage the blood of the fetus if it is Rhesus positive.

Compatibility

In a blood transfusion, if the blood given to a patient (**recipient**) from a **donor** contains a factor in the cells to which the patient's (recipient's) blood serum will react, the donor's blood will be destroyed, causing clumping together of the red cells (agglutination) which can be fatal. Therefore blood is normally 'cross-matched' for compatibility before transfusion is given. In extreme emergencies, the 'universal donor' group is given, i.e. O Rhesus -ve, before any investigations are done.

In normal circumstances the same group as the recipient is given.

- Group AB Rh +ve is the **universal recipient**.
- Group O Rh -ve is the **universal donor**.

ABBREVIATIONS

AIDS	acquired immunodeficiency syndrome
ALL	acute lymphocytic leukaemia
AML	acute myeloid leukaemia
APT	activated prothrombin time
APPT	activated partial thromboplastin time
BUN	blood urea nitrogen
CLL	chronic lymphocytic leukaemia
CML	chronic myeloid leukaemia
CO₂	carbon dioxide
ESR	erythrocyte sedimentation rate
FBC	full blood count
Hb	haemoglobin (pigmented protein which carries oxygen)
HDL	high density lipoprotein
Ig	immunoglobulin
INR	international normalised ratio (prothrombin time)

LDL	low density lipoprotein
MCH	mean corpuscular haemoglobin
MCHC	mean corpuscular haemoglobin concentration
MCV	mean corpuscular volume
O$_2$	oxygen
PCV	packed cell volume
RBC	red blood count
TIBC	total iron-binding capacity
WBC	white blood count
WBC & diff.	white blood count and different percentages present

UNITS USED IN BIOCHEMISTRY

SI	international system (Système International)
IU or U	international unit
mmol	millimole
mmol/l	millimole per litre
nmol	nanomole
µmol	micromole
µg	microgram
g	gram

TERMINOLOGY

Ery-, Erythro-	red
Haem-, Haemato-	stem for blood
Leuco-	white
Thrombo-	clot
Coagulation	clotting of blood
Gamma-globulin	plasma proteins which include antibodies
Haemostasis	stopping bleeding
Immunoglobulin	plasma proteins which are antibodies

(see also pathology section)

DISEASES AND DISORDERS

Agranulocytosis	large decrease in number of white granulocytes (cells which fight against infection).
Anaemia	amount of oxygen carrying capacity is reduced due to either too few red blood cells or too little haemoglobin.
Epistaxis	nose-bleed.
Haemolysis	destruction of blood cells.

Haemophilia A	hereditary disease caused by lack of clotting factor (VIII) in the blood.
Haemophilia B	hereditary disease caused by lack of clotting factor (IX) in the blood.
HIV	human immunodeficiency virus.
Hyper-cholesterolaemia	raised blood cholesterol (lipid or fat) levels.
Hyperlipidaemia	raised blood fat levels.
Hypochromic anaemia	anaemia associated with pale, small red cells due to insufficient iron.
Infectious mononucleosis	glandular fever - increase of white cells called monocytes present in blood.
Leucocytosis	a normal increase of white blood cells in response to infection.
Leucopenia	a decrease in the number of white blood cells in the blood.
Leukaemia	a cancer of the blood - abnormal white cells increase.
Pernicious anaemia	inability of body to manufacture normal red blood cells due to a missing factor.
Polycythaemia	too many red and other blood cells present in the blood.
Sickle-cell anaemia	anaemia associated with people of African ethnic origin, red cells have sickle shape.
Thalassaemia	anaemia associated with people of Mediterranean origin.

PROCEDURES AND EQUIPMENT

Cryoprecipitate	use of subartic temperatures to separate required factors from blood.
Paul-Bunnell test	blood test for glandular fever.
Plasmapheresis	taking blood from a donor, removing the required factor and returning the remainder to the donor's circulation.

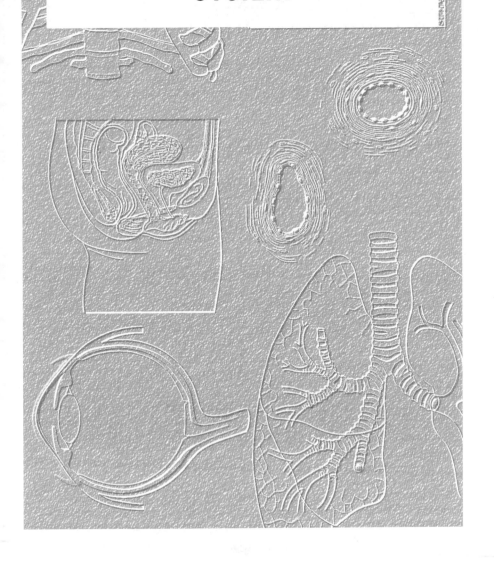

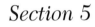
Section 5

THE CARDIOVASCULAR SYSTEM

STRUCTURE AND FUNCTION

This consists of the heart and blood vessels, and the transportation of blood throughout the body.

Organs forming the system are the:
- **Heart**
- **Blood vessels**

THE HEART

Structure

This is a hollow muscular organ, the size of the owner's fist, situated in the **mediastinal space** (between the lungs) of the **thoracic** (chest) cavity. It is tilted to the left and its base rests upon the diaphragm.

It is composed of three layers of tissue:

Pericardium	a specialised fibrous sac, lined with serous membrane, covering the heart and preventing friction.
Myocardium	composed of cardiac muscle forming the chambers and septum.
Endocardium	a smooth endothelial lining which also forms the valves.

The heart is a double pump. It consists of two thin-walled upper chambers known as **atria** and two thick-walled lower chambers known as **ventricles**, the left ventricle having the thickest wall. It is divided into left and right sides by a muscular septum. Blood contained in the left chambers has no communication with that in the right (see Figure 20).

Valves of the heart

The upper and lower chambers are separated by non-return valves which prevent the backflow of blood - the **tricuspid valve** between the right chambers and the **bicuspid** or **mitral** valve between the left chambers.

Specialised nerve supply to the heart

The **vagus nerve** supplies the heart as well as fibres from the **sympathetic chain** of the **autonomic nervous system** (ANS) (see Section 13).

There are also specialised areas of nerve fibres within the heart muscle. These are the:

- **sinu-atrial** node in the wall of the right atrium (**pacemaker**);
- **atrioventricular node** in the wall at the junction of the atria and ventricles;
- **bundle of His** in the ventricular septum of the heart.

Function

The cardiac cycle

The two upper chambers (atria) receive blood from the veins and, on contraction, force blood through the valves into the lower chambers (ventricles). This impulse is controlled by the sinu-atrial node. As the atria relax, blood is automatically sucked in from the attached blood vessels to refill these chambers.

As the atria relax, so the ventricles contract (at an impulse from the atrioventricular node, conducted down through the bundle of His), pumping blood into the attached arteries through one-way valves which guard their openings. The ventricles relax and the cycle recommences.

Blood flow

The right side of the heart contains deoxygenated blood, returned from the body via veins; the left side contains oxygenated blood returned from the lungs where gases have been exchanged. The left ventricle, the thickest walled chamber, pumps blood to the body via the main artery, the **aorta**.

Heart sounds

Two sounds, which are produced by the closing of valves, can be clearly heard during the cardiac cycle.

'**Lubb**' a long, dull sound is produced at the closing of the valves between the upper and lower chambers of the heart (**atrioventricular valves**), whilst '**dup**', a sharp, short sound is produced by the closing of the valves guarding the arteries arising from the ventricles (the **pulmonary** and **aortic valves**).

It is these sounds which are known as the heart sounds. Abnormality may be caused by disease of the heart valves as in cases of **rheumatic fever** and the sounds produced are then known as '**murmurs**'.

BLOOD VESSELS

These form a completely closed system which transports blood, containing various substances, to and from the heart via all the tissues of the body.

They consist of:
- **Arteries** (see Figure 21)
- **Veins** (see Figure 22)
- **Capillaries**

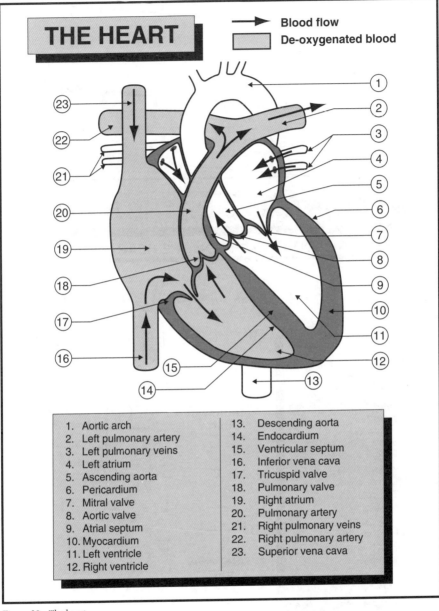

Blood flow
De-oxygenated blood

THE HEART

1. Aortic arch
2. Left pulmonary artery
3. Left pulmonary veins
4. Left atrium
5. Ascending aorta
6. Pericardium
7. Mitral valve
8. Aortic valve
9. Atrial septum
10. Myocardium
11. Left ventricle
12. Right ventricle
13. Descending aorta
14. Endocardium
15. Ventricular septum
16. Inferior vena cava
17. Tricuspid valve
18. Pulmonary valve
19. Right atrium
20. Pulmonary artery
21. Right pulmonary veins
22. Right pulmonary artery
23. Superior vena cava

Figure 20 - The heart.

Arteries

Arteries, varying in size, are vessels travelling from the heart and (apart from the **pulmonary artery** travelling to the lungs which contains de-oxygenated blood) contain oxygenated blood. They contain muscle and elastic tissue in their walls to allow for contraction and relaxation with the contraction of the heart. They have a very smooth lining to prevent clotting. The smallest arteries are known as **arterioles**.

Veins

There are more veins than arteries in the body. Veins, varying in size, carry deoxygenated blood (apart from the **pulmonary veins** containing oxygenated blood) returning to the heart. They have a similar structure to arteries, but the walls are thinner and much less elastic (Figure 23). If a vein is cut it collapses, but an artery remains open and spurts blood rhythmically. Veins possess one-way valves to prevent backflow of blood. It is these which become damaged in the condition of **varicose veins**. The smallest veins are known as **venules**.

Capillaries

These are fine, hair-like vessels, consisting of one-cell-thick coats. It is from these structures, because they are only one cell thick, that fluid (**tissue fluid**) containing oxygen, nutrients and other substances, is able to flow into the tissues, so supplying the individual cells with their requirements.

These blood vessels are the only ones where substances are able to leave the blood stream. Large proteins remain behind in the blood vessels, as they are too large to pass through the capillary walls. These proteins enable some of the fluid to

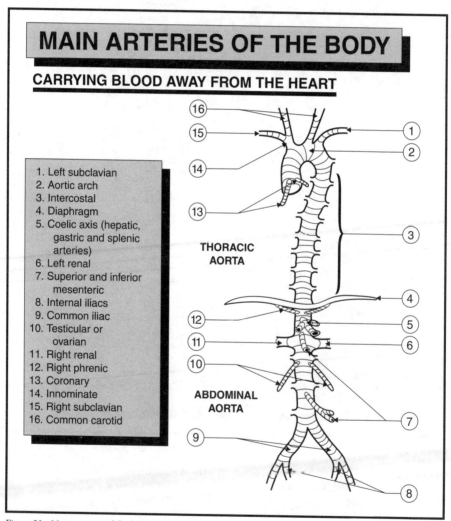

MAIN ARTERIES OF THE BODY

CARRYING BLOOD AWAY FROM THE HEART

1. Left subclavian
2. Aortic arch
3. Intercostal
4. Diaphragm
5. Coelic axis (hepatic, gastric and splenic arteries)
6. Left renal
7. Superior and inferior mesenteric
8. Internal iliacs
9. Common iliac
10. Testicular or ovarian
11. Right renal
12. Right phrenic
13. Coronary
14. Innominate
15. Right subclavian
16. Common carotid

THORACIC AORTA

ABDOMINAL AORTA

Figure 21 - Main arteries of the body.

be attracted back into the venous capillaries by **osmosis**. The remaining fluid (**lymph**) is returned to the circulation via the lymphatic system (see Section 6).

Main blood vessels:

Aorta	main artery of the body, stems from the left ventricle to supply the body with oxygenated blood.
Pulmonary artery	takes blood to the lungs for oxygenation and removal of carbon dioxide.
Superior vena cava **Inferior vena cava**	main veins of the body. returning blood from the body to the right atrium.
Pulmonary veins	returns oxygenated blood to the left side of the heart for distribution to the body via the aorta.

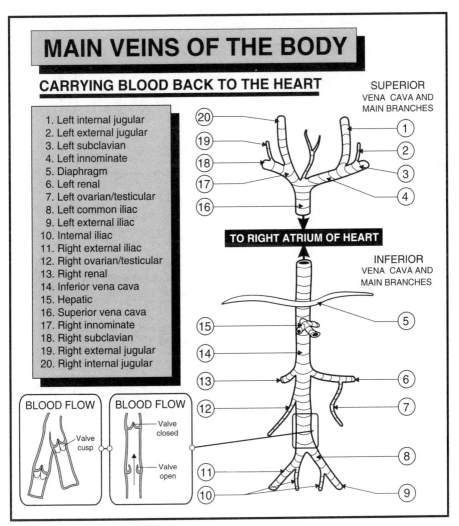

MAIN VEINS OF THE BODY

CARRYING BLOOD BACK TO THE HEART

SUPERIOR VENA CAVA AND MAIN BRANCHES

1. Left internal jugular
2. Left external jugular
3. Left subclavian
4. Left innominate
5. Diaphragm
6. Left renal
7. Left ovarian/testicular
8. Left common iliac
9. Left external iliac
10. Internal iliac
11. Right external iliac
12. Right ovarian/testicular
13. Right renal
14. Inferior vena cava
15. Hepatic
16. Superior vena cava
17. Right innominate
18. Right subclavian
19. Right external jugular
20. Right internal jugular

TO RIGHT ATRIUM OF HEART

INFERIOR VENA CAVA AND MAIN BRANCHES

BLOOD FLOW — Valve cusp

BLOOD FLOW — Valve closed — Valve open

Figure 22 - Main veins of the body.

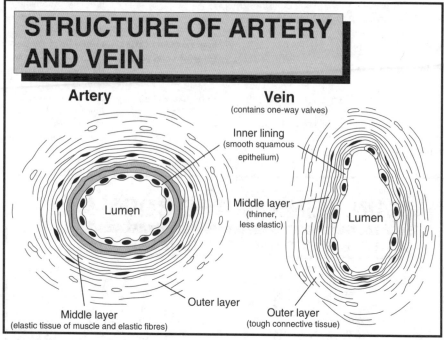

STRUCTURE OF ARTERY AND VEIN

Artery

Vein
(contains one-way valves)

Inner lining
(smooth squamous
epithelium)

Lumen

Middle layer
(thinner,
less elastic)

Lumen

Outer layer

Middle layer
(elastic tissue of muscle and elastic fibres)

Outer layer
(tough connective tissue)

Figure 23 - Structure of artery and vein.

BLOOD CIRCULATION

Systemic supplies the main body; the main artery is the **aorta** from which other large arteries arise; all organs have their own blood supply.

Pulmonary supplies the lungs for oxygenation of the blood and removal of carbon dioxide - oxygenated blood is returned to the left atrium.

Portal supplies the liver and is concerned with the transport of food substances from the intestine for assimilation by the liver; the liver has two blood supplies from the hepatic artery and the portal vein.

BLOOD PRESSURE (ARTERIAL)

This is the force, or pressure, that the blood is exerting against the walls of the blood vessels in which it is contained. This pressure varies during the cardiac cycle.

Systolic pressure

This is the pressure felt when the ventricles of the heart are contracting and pumping blood through the arteries via the main aorta. This is also known as the **systole**. It is the higher reading.

Diastolic pressure

This is the pressure felt when the heart chambers are at rest as the heart relaxes. This is also known as the **diastole**. It is the lower reading.

Factors affecting normal blood pressure:

- Cardiac output - the pumping of the heart.
- Volume of the blood circulating.
- Peripheral resistance of the blood vessels - the **calibre** (diameter) of small arteries away from the centre of the body - this is also affected by hardening and narrowing caused by age and fatty deposits (**atherosclerosis**).
- Elastic recoil of large arteries.
- Viscosity (thickness) of the blood.

PULSE

This is a wave of distension and recoil, which can be felt in the wall of an artery as it passes over a bone near the surface of the body. It reflects the pressure transmitted from the aorta at the beating of the heart.

Normal pulse range (number of beats per minute)

In the newborn	140
Infants	120
Children at 10 years.	80 - 90
Adults	60 - 80 (average 72)

Emotion, exercise, age and health will all affect the pulse rate.

ABBREVIATIONS

AS	aortic stenosis
ASD	atrial septum defect
ASHD	arteriosclerotic heart disease
AST*	aspartate transaminase (cardiac enzyme)
BP	blood pressure
CABG	coronary artery bypass graft
CABS	coronary artery bypass surgery
CAD	coronary artery disease
CCF	congestive cardiac failure
CCU	coronary care unit
CHF	congestive heart failure
CPK*	creatine phosphokinase (cardiac enzyme)
CPR	cardiopulmonary resuscitation
CVP	central venous pressure
CVS	cardiovascular system
DVT	deep vein thrombosis
ECG	electrocardiogram (records the electrical impulses of the beating of the heart muscle)
GOT*	glutamic-oxaloacetic transaminase (cardiac enzyme)
HI	hypodermic injection
HS	heart sounds
ICU	intensive care unit
IM	intramuscular injection
ITU	intensive therapy unit
IV	intravenous injection
LD*	lactate dehydrogenase (cardiac enzyme)
PAT	paroxysmal atrial tachycardia
PTCA	percutaneous transluminal coronary angioplasty
PVC	premature ventricular contraction
TMR	transmyocardial revascularisation
VSD	ventricular septal defect

* These enzymes also indicate metabolism of other organs

TERMINOLOGY

Angi/o	stem for blood vessel.
Arteri/o	stem for artery.
Cardi/o (Coron/o)	stem for heart.
Phleb/o (Ven/o)	stem for vein.
Blood pressure	normally referring to the force of blood felt against the artery walls on the contraction and relaxation of the left ventricle (chamber of heart), measured in millimetres of mercury (mmHg).
Cardiology	study of the heart.
Diastole	the relaxation phase of the heart cycle where chambers fill with blood - this is the lower reading of blood pressure.
Pulse	a wave of distension and relaxation felt where an artery crosses a bone near the surface of the body.
Sinus rhythm	the heart beating in normal rhythm.
Systole	the contraction phase of the cardiac cycle - the force felt when the left ventricle contracts, forcing blood through the aorta to supply the body with its blood supply.
Vascular	referring to blood vessels.

DISEASES AND DISORDERS

Aneurysm   a weakness in the wall of an artery (can cause ballooning and rupture).

Angina pectoris   pain in the chest and left arm caused by insufficient blood to the heart muscle, usually on exertion or excitement.

Angioma   tumour of blood vessels, usually capillaries.

Arrhythmia   abnormal rhythm of the heart.

Arteriosclerosis   hardening of an artery.

Arteritis   inflammation of an artery.

Atheroma   fatty deposits in the wall of an artery.

Atherosclerosis   narrowing (with fatty deposits) and hardening of an artery.

Atrial fibrillation   disorder of the heart beat, no co-ordination between atria and ventricles.

Bradycardia   an abnormally slow heart beat.

Cardiac arrest   cessation of the heart beat.

Cardiac asthma   breathlessness caused by right-sided failure of the heart, usually at night.

Carditis   inflammation of the heart.

Coronary occlusion   a sudden blocking of an artery supplying the heart muscle, e.g. thrombosis (formation of a blood clot).

Coronary thrombosis   a blocking of an artery by a blood clot in the coronary (heart) circulation.

Cyanosis   blueness of the skin and mucous membranes due to lack of oxygen.

Diastolic murmur   abnormal sound heard during relaxation phase of the cardiac cycle.

Dyspnoea   laboured or difficult breathing.

Embolism   sudden obstruction of a blood vessel by an embolus.

Embolus   a detached and travelling particle of fat, air or blood clot.

Endocarditis   inflammation of the lining of the heart (endocardium).

Fibrillation   a quivering of the heart chambers, an ineffective action of pumping blood.

Haemorrhoids   varicose veins of the rectum.

Hypertension (hyperpiesis)   high blood pressure

Intermittent claudication   painful condition of the leg caused by lack of blood supply.

Mitral incompetence   disordered function of the mitral valve of the heart (between the left chambers of the heart).

Mitral stenosis   narrowing of the mitral valve.

Myocardial infarct   death (necrosis) of a wedge-shaped area of heart tissue when the artery supplying it becomes blocked.

Myocarditis   inflammation of the muscle of the heart.

Oedema   excess fluid in the tissues.

Palpitations   rapid forceful beating of heart of which the patient is aware.

Pancarditis   inflammation of all structures of the heart.

Patent ductus arteriosus   failure of the ductus arteriosus (artery bypassing lungs in fetus) to close at birth.

Pericarditis   inflammation of the outside covering of the heart.

Phlebitis   inflammation of a vein.

Phlebolith	stone in a vein (calcium deposits).
Pulmonary stenosis	narrowing of the valve between the right ventricle and pulmonary artery.
Systolic murmur	abnormal sound heard during contraction phase of cardiac cycle.
Tachycardia	a rapid heart beat.
Thrombophlebitis	inflammation of the wall of a vein causing a blood clot to form (thrombus).
Thrombosis	a condition where a thrombus has formed.
Thrombus	a blood clot in a blood vessel.
Varices	varicose veins.
Varicose veins	presence of thickened and twisted veins caused by incompetent valves.
Ventricular fibrillation	a quivering of the ventricles of the heart instead of contracting forcefully.

PROCEDURES AND EQUIPMENT

Angiocardiography	demonstration of heart and major blood vessels using an opaque medium injected into the circulation.
Angiogram	special X-ray of arteries using radio-opaque medium (dye which shows up in X-rays).
Angioplasty	reshaping or forming a blood vessel.
Aortograph	recording of a pulse on a graph demonstration of aorta by use of opaque medium.
Arteriotomy	cutting into an artery.
Auscultation	listening to sounds for diagnostic purposes, usually with a stethoscope.
Cardiac catheterisation	a fine hollow tube (catheter) is inserted into heart chamber to measure gases and pressure/radio-opaque dye is introduced.
Defibrillation	restoring the heart rhythm to normal sinus rhythm by means of electrical shock from defibrillator.
ECG	see abbreviations.
Endarterectomy	surgical removal of deposits (e.g. fat, blood clots) from the lining of arteries.
Exercise tolerance test	test on the heart during exercise (ECG).
Haemorrhoidectomy	surgical removal of haemorrhoids.
Injection of varicose veins	treatment of varicose veins - an injection is given of a substance which will cause the vein to sclerose, i.e. seal up.
Intravascular thrombolysis	an agent which destroys/dissolves clots is infused into the blood vessels to clear a blood clot (thrombus).
Ligation of varicose veins	surgically tying off parts of a varicose vein to divert the blood supply through healthier veins.
Pacemaker	referring to: *a)* an artificial implant of an electrical mechanism to replace the damaged sinu-atrial node. *b)* the sinu-atrial node of specialised nerve tissue in the wall of the right atrium which initiates the contraction of the heart.
Percutaneous transluminal coronary angioplasty	a procedure where an occluded (blocked) blood vessel is dilated using a ballon catheter; guidance is provided by a monitor which shows the position of the catheter within the body by fluoroscopy.

Phlebotomy	cutting into a vein.	in order to stimulate
Phonocardiography	the heart sounds of	growth of new blood
	the cardiac cycle (con-	vessels to increase
	traction and relaxation	blood supply to dam-
	of the chambers) are	aged heart muscle
	displayed as graphic **Valvectomy**	surgical removal of a
	images on a monitor;	valve.
	an ECG is displayed **Valvotomy**	cutting into a valve, by
	simultaneously	custom referring to
Sphygmomanometer	instrument used for	the heart.
	measuring blood pres- **Varicotomy**	cutting into a varicose
	sure.	vein.
Stethoscope	instrument used for **Venepuncture**	insertion of a needle
	listening to sounds of	into a vein.
	the body. **Venesection**	cutting down into a
Stripping of	surgical procedure	vein for purposes of
varicose veins	where varicose veins	transfusion or inser-
	are removed.	tion of drugs.
Transmyocardial	a procedure where **Venogram**	X-ray of a vein
revascularisation	small holes are made	using an opaque
	in the cardiac muscle	medium.

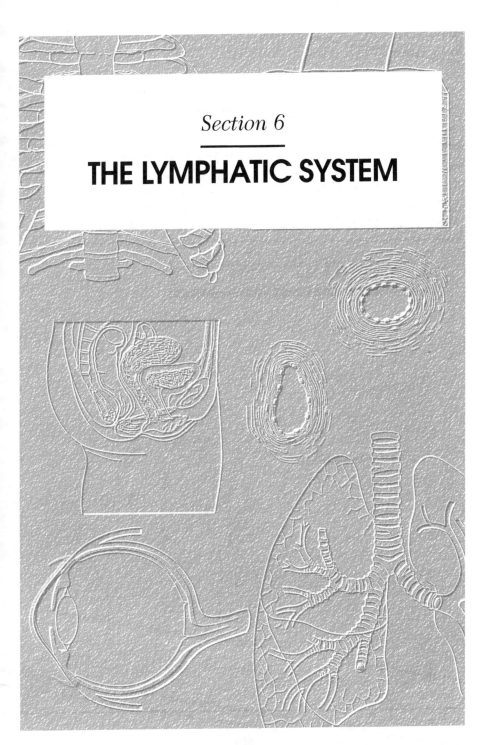

Section 6

THE LYMPHATIC SYSTEM

FUNCTION

The lymphatic system is a transport and defence system.

Lymph is the remains of **tissue fluid** after it has passed through the tissues from the capillaries and given up its nutrients and gases to the cells. It has gathered waste products and is returned to the circulation via the lymphatic system.

STRUCTURE

It consists of the following (see Figure 24):

- Lymph.
- Lymph capillaries.
- Lymph vessels.
- Lymph nodes or glands, superficial and deep.
- Main lymph ducts.
- Specialised lymph glands.

Lymph capillaries

These are similar in structure to the blood capillaries, but start in the tissue spaces and are open-ended tubes; they are not continuous.

Lymph vessels

These are similar in structure to veins, but have many more valves in their walls giving a beaded appearance.

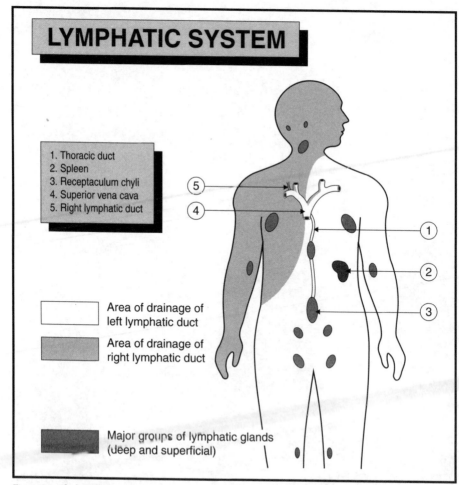

LYMPHATIC SYSTEM

1. Thoracic duct
2. Spleen
3. Receptaculum chyli
4. Superior vena cava
5. Right lymphatic duct

Area of drainage of left lymphatic duct

Area of drainage of right lymphatic duct

Major groups of lymphatic glands (deep and superficial)

Figure 24 - The lymphatic system.

Lymph nodes or glands

These act as filters between the returning lymph fluid and the vessels, trapping debris and bacteria, and are part of the defence system of the body. Cancer cells are also filtered here, but unfortunately some of these cells manage to reach the main blood stream and secondary deposits of these malignant cells occur in distant tissues (**metastases**).

They also manufacture some types of white blood cells (lymphocytes and monocytes).

Main lymph ducts

These consist of:

- **Right lymphatic duct**
- **Thoracic duct**

The right lymphatic duct drains lymph from the right upper trunk, head and right arm.

The thoracic duct receives lymph from the rest of the body. It also receives fat absorbed from the **ileum** of the small intestine.

The contents of both of these ducts empty into the main veins of the body for circulation.

Specialised lymph glands

These include:

- **Tonsils** and **adenoids**.
- **Peyer's patches** in the ileum.
- **Appendix** in the large intestine.
- **Spleen** in the abdominal cavity.

They act as defence mechanisms and also manufacture some types of white blood cells (lymphocytes).

Peyer's patches become infected in cases of **typhoid fever**.

The **spleen** also controls the volume and quality of blood circulating, destroys worn out red blood cells and produces antibodies.

TERMINOLOGY

Lymph/o	stem for lymph
Aden/o	stem for gland (any)
Splen/o	stem for spleen
Antibodies	produced by lymphocytes, they help to overcome infection.
Antitoxins	these neutralise poisons produced by micro-organisms.
Lymph	fluid draining from the tissues to be returned to the circulation.
Lymphocyte	white blood cell which is manufactured in lymphatic tissue and fights infection by producing antibodies and antitoxins.

DISEASES AND DISORDERS

Adenitis	inflammation of a gland.
Adenoma	tumour of glands.
Anasarca	widely spread oedema.
Ascites	free fluid in the peritoneal cavity.
Hodgkin's disease	malignant disease of the lymphatic system caused by a virus.
Infectious mononucleosis	glandular fever.
Lymphadenoma	tumour of lymph gland.
Lymphangitis	inflammation of lymph vessels.
Lymphocythaemia	excessive number of lymphocytes in the blood.
Lymphocytopenia	deficiency of lymphocytes in the blood.
Metastasis (**pl. metastases**)	secondary deposit(s) of malignant cells from a primary tumour or source (usually through the lymph channels).
Oedema	free fluid in the tissues (fluid is not draining back to circulation).
Splenitis	inflammation of the spleen.
Splenomegaly	enlargement of the spleen.

PROCEDURES AND EQUIPMENT

Adenectomy	surgical removal of a gland.
Lymphangiogram	special X-ray of the lymph vessels with an opaque dye.

Paracentesis abdominis	drawing off of free fluid from the abdominal/peritoneal cavity.	**Paracentesis tympani**	drawing off of fluid from the middle ear.
Paracentesis thoracis	drawing off of fluid from the chest cavity (thorax).	**Splenectomy**	surgical removal of the spleen.
		Splenogram	special X-ray of the spleen using opaque dye.

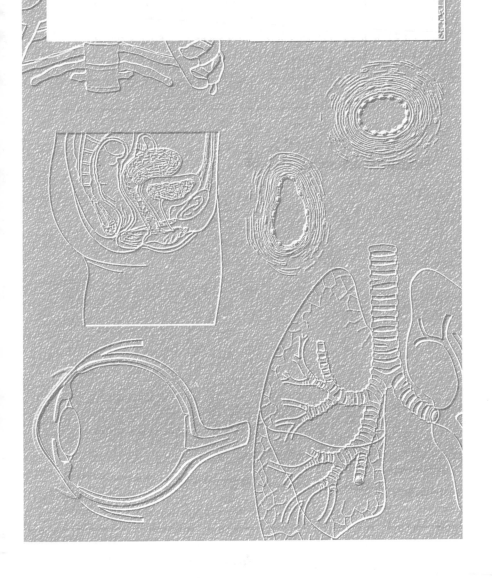

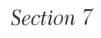

Section 7

THE RESPIRATORY SYSTEM

FUNCTION

This system is concerned with the vital function of external respiration, the exchange of gases - taking in oxygen from the air and the excretion of carbon dioxide and water vapour as waste products.

STRUCTURE

This consists of the following organs:

- **Nose**
- **Nasopharynx** } upper respiratory tract
- **Larynx**
- **Trachea**
- Two **bronchi**
- **Bronchioles**
- **Alveoli** } lower respiratory tract
- **Lungs**

Nose

The nose is made up of bone and cartilage and is connected to the **sinuses** (spaces of air). Its function is to receive, moisten, warm and filter air. It is also the organ of the sense of smell which is closely linked with taste (see Section 14).

Pharynx

This extends from the back of the nose to the larynx, and the nasopharynx is the area at the back of the nose. The **eustachian tube** from the middle ear enters here. Both air and food pass through the pharynx.

Larynx (see Figure 25)

This is also known as the voice box as it contains the vocal cords (Figure 26), two delicate folds of membrane which vibrate to produce sound.

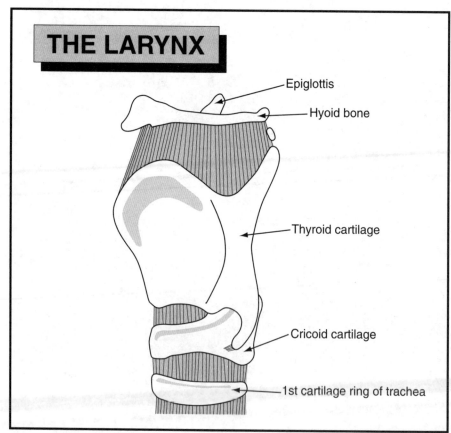

THE LARYNX

Epiglottis

Hyoid bone

Thyroid cartilage

Cricoid cartilage

1st cartilage ring of trachea

Figure 25 - Larynx (lateral view).

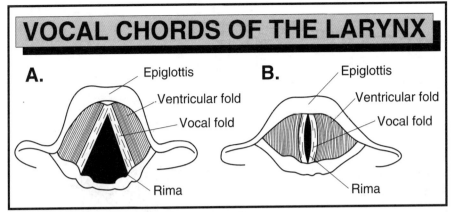

VOCAL CHORDS OF THE LARYNX

A.
Epiglottis
Ventricular fold
Vocal fold
Rima

B.
Epiglottis
Ventricular fold
Vocal fold
Rima

Figure 26 - Vocal chords of larynx (A - relaxed, B - in speech).

The larynx is composed of several irregular-shaped cartilages:

- **epiglottis**
- **thyroid cartilage**
- **two arytenoid cartilages**
- **cricoid cartilage**

The thyroid cartilage, also known as the **Adam's apple** is found at the anterior of the larynx. The cricoid cartilage is shaped like a signet ring, whilst the arytenoid cartilages are attached to the vocal cords.

The entrance to the larynx, known as the **glottis**, is guarded by a flap of cartilage called the **epiglottis**. This structure prevents food or fluid passing into the air passages. This occurs automatically by a reflex action when the person is conscious. **However, in a state of unconsciousness this reflex does not occur and blockage of the airway can easily result**.

Trachea

This is known as the **windpipe** and is continuous with the larynx and extends to the bronchi. It is composed of several C-shaped rings of cartilage, which keep the structure open to allow air to pass down into the lungs.

Bronchi

These are two short tubes, the right and left bronchi, continuous with the trachea and containing cartilage and muscle. The bronchi enter the lung at an area known as the **hilum**. The bronchi divide into numerous branches known as **bronchioles** - smaller tubes of similar structure

to the bronchi, but which contain more muscle tissue in their walls. These take air to the delicate air sacs at their terminations known as **alveoli**.

Lungs

These are two pink, spongy, cone-shaped organs lying in the thoracic cavity (the chest), one either side of the heart and great blood vessels. The base of each lung rests upon the **diaphragm** and the apex lies just below the level of the **clavicle** (collar-bone). The right and left lungs consist of lobes, covered in a serous membrane known as the **pleura**. The right lung, which is larger, has three lobes, the left lung has two. These are further divided into **lobules**, each being complete in itself, and including blood vessels, lymphatic vessels, elastic connective tissue, bronchioles and alveoli (Figure 27).

Alveoli

These are tiny, delicate, one-cell-thick air sacs surrounded by a capillary network from the pulmonary circulation. This membrane is moist and it is only here that the exchange of gases occurs. All other parts of the respiratory tract or airway convey air to the air sacs for this vital purpose.

VENTILATION

This consists of **inspiration** (breathing in) and **expiration** (breathing out). The muscles of respiration are essential for this proces; these are the diaphragm and the **intercostal muscles** (between the ribs).

Inspiration

The chest cavity expands as the muscles of

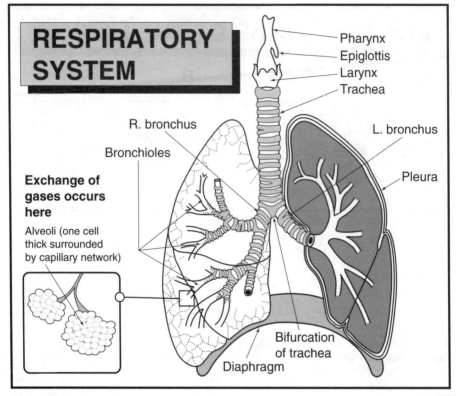

RESPIRATORY SYSTEM

Pharynx
Epiglottis
Larynx
Trachea

R. bronchus

L. bronchus

Bronchioles

Pleura

Exchange of gases occurs here

Alveoli (one cell thick surrounded by capillary network)

Bifurcation of trachea

Diaphragm

Figure 27 - Respiratory system.

respiration contract, swinging the rib cage out and the diaphragm down. The action is similar to a pair of bellows and air containing oxygen is sucked in through the nose/mouth to fill the expanding lungs.

Expiration

When these muscles relax it has the opposite function to inspiration, decreasing the size of the chest cavity and forcing out expired air through the airway, removing waste gases of carbon dioxide and water vapour. Figures 28 and 29 show instruments designed for measuring peak expiratory flow.

AIR CONTENT

Inspired air contains 21% oxygen and 0.04% carbon dioxide.

Expired air contains 17% oxygen and 4% carbon dioxide.

In **cardiopulmonary resuscitation**, the presence of oxygen in the expired air provides suffi-

cient oxygen for the patient's requirements. The higher level of carbon dioxide present can, in certain situations, also stimulate the **respiratory centre** in the brain to start spontaneous respiration.

RESPIRATION

Breathing is an automatic process, although it can be controlled by the will. It is controlled by the respiratory centre in the brain which responds to the level of carbon dioxide in the blood. Oxygen is vital for every cell and the brain cells have the greatest requirement. If they do not receive a supply of oxygen for three to four minutes brain damage will occur and death will usually result. If the person is resuscitated after this time period, there is likely to be permanent damage to the brain.

Exchange of gases

Pressure of oxygen in inspired air in the air sacs is high while the oxygen pressure within the capillary blood surrounding these sacs is low.

54

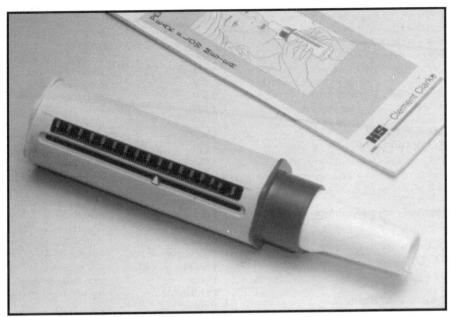

Figure 28 - Miniwright standard range peak flow meter (for adults). Reproduced with kind permission from Clement Clarke International Ltd.

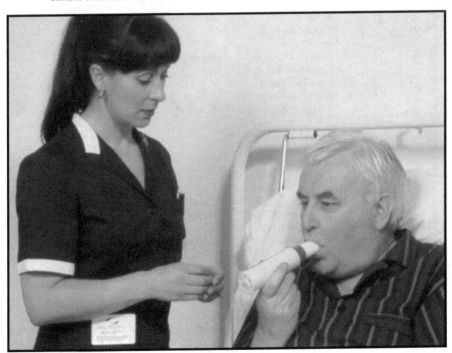

Figure 29 - Peak flow meter in use. Reproduced with kind permission from Clement Clarke International Ltd.

Therefore the oxygen passes through the membrane into the blood, combining with the haemoglobin of the red cells to be carried back to the heart for distribution to the body.

Pressure of carbon dioxide in the air sacs is low, while the pressure of it within the capillary blood is high. Therefore carbon dioxide passes through the membrane into the air sac and is breathed out of the lungs on expiration.

Respiration rate

The rate of respiration will vary with the individual, increasing with exercise, emotion, certain diseases and fever.

Normal rate per minute

Newborn (first four weeks)	40
Infants (four weeks to one year)	30
Children (up to five years)	24
Adults	12 - 18

ABBREVIATIONS

AP	artificial pneumothorax
COAD	chronic obstructive airway disease
COLD	chronic obstructive lung disease
COPD	chronic obstructive pulmonary disease
CPR	cardiopulmonary resuscitation
FB	foreign body
IPPB	intermittent positive pressure breathing
LRTI	lower respiratory tract infection
PCP	*Pneumocystis carinii* pneumonia (associated with AIDS)
PE	pulmonary embolism
PEFR	peak expiratory flow rate (see vital capacity)
PND	paroxysmal nocturnal dyspnoea
RD	respiratory disease
RDS	respiratory distress syndrome
SMR	submucous resection (altering the structure of the nasal septum, i.e. cartilage division, or correcting crooked septum)
SOB	shortness of breath
Ts & As	tonsillectomy and adenoidectomy
TB	tuberculosis
URI	upper respiratory infection
URTI	upper respiratory tract infection
VC	vital capacity

TERMINOLOGY

Bronch/o	stem for bronchus(i).
Laryng/o	stem for larynx (voice box).
Nas/o	stem for nose.
Pharyng/o	stem for throat.
Pneum/o (pneumon/o)	stems for lungs.
Pnoe-	stem for breathing.
Pulmon/o	stem for lung.
Rhin/o	stem for nose.
Tonsill/o	stem for tonsils.
Trache/o	stem for trachea (windpipe).
Adenoids	specialised lymphatic tissue behind the nose (naso-pharynx).
Bronchioles	the smallest tubes of the lungs between the bronchi and the alveoli.
Epiglottis	flap of cartilage which guards the entrance of the glottis to prevent food being inhaled into the larynx (reflex action in the conscious person).
Nasal	referring to the nose.
Pleura	membrane covering lobes of lungs.
Vital capacity	amount of air which can be breathed out on a forced expiration following a forced inspiration (as on a peak expiratory flow meter).

DISEASES AND DISORDERS

Apnoea	cessation of breathing.
Asphyxia	lack of oxygen in the

blood and thus the tissues.

Asthma   inflammatory disease of the bronchial tubes due to hypersensitivity to foreign proteins (allergy) resulting in narrowing of airway as the result of bronchial constriction.

Atelectasis   failure of the lungs to expand, e.g. at birth, or collapse of the alveoli (air sacs).

Bronchiectasis   over dilatation of the bronchioles due to fibrous tissue.

Bronchitis   inflammation of the bronchial tubes.

Cheyne–Stokes respiration   irregular breathing with periods of cessation of breathing (apnoea) and over-breathing (hyperventilation); this is due to change in pH of the blood passing through respiratory centre in the brain resulting from levels of urea build up in body as kidneys fail - this usually results in death.

Cor pulmonale   right ventricular heart failure caused by lung disease

Coryza   the common cold.

Crêpitations   fine crackling which can be heard.

Cyanosis   blueness of the skin and mucous membranes due to lack of oxygen.

Dyspnoea   difficulty in breathing.

Epiglottitis   inflammation of the epiglottis.

Epistaxis   nose-bleed.

Haemoptysis   coughing up of blood from the lungs, usually bright red and frothy.

Hypoxia   insufficient oxygen in the blood.

Laryngeal stridor   harsh sounds on inspiration - can be due to spasm.

Laryngitis   inflammation of the larynx.

Laryngostenosis   constriction (narrowing) of the larynx.

Lobectomy   surgical removal of a lobe of lung.

Nasal polyp   pedunculated tumour of the lining of the nose (tumour with a stalk).

Orthopnoea   only able to breath when sitting upright.

Pharyngitis   inflammation of the throat (pharynx).

Pleurisy (pleuritis)   inflammation of the pleura, with effusion, producing fluid.

Pneumonia (pneumonitis)   inflammation of the lungs.

Pneumothorax   air in the pleural cavity causing collapse of lung.

Pulmonary emphysema   abnormal distension of the alveoli (air sacs) of the lungs in chronic respiratory disease, e.g. bronchiectasis.

Pulmonary empyema   presence of pus in the pleural cavity.

Râle   abnormal rattling sound heard - present in bronchitis and pneumonia.

Rhinitis   inflammation of the nose.

Rhinorrhoea   discharge from the nose.

Rhonchi   abnormal sounds in the bronchial tubes on listening with a stethoscope (auscultation).

Sinusitis   inflammation of the lining of the cavities of the nasal and skull bones.

Spontaneous pneumothorax   collapse of the lung spontaneously.

Stertorous   noisy breathing, as in snoring, due to obstruction, e.g.

tongue falling to back of throat.

Tachypnoea rapid breathing, as in pneumonia.

Tonsillitis inflammation of the tonsils (specialised lymphoid tissue).

Tracheitis inflammation of the trachea.

Tuberculosis an infection of the lung or other organs by the bacteria *tubercule bacillus* (unfortunately this is increasing)

PROCEDURES AND EQUIPMENT

Adenoidectomy surgical removal of the adenoids.

Antral puncture puncture of the antrum (sinus) in the maxillary bone of the face through the nose in order to drain pus and washout the cavity (antral washout).

Artificial pneumothorax collapse of the lung by the deliberate introduction of air into the chest cavity.

Auscultation listening to sounds with a stethoscope.

Bronchogram special X-ray of the bronchial tubes using an opaque medium.

Bronchoscopy examination of the bronchi with a lighted instrument.

Heaf test skin test for tuberculosis.

Intubation introduction of a tube into air passages to allow air into the lungs (as in anaesthesia).

Kveim test skin test for sarcoidosis.

Laryngectomy surgical removal of the larynx.

Laryngoscope a lighted instrument used for examination of the larynx.

Laryngoscopy examination of the larynx with a lighted instrument.

Lobectomy surgical removal of a lobe of the lung.

Mantoux test skin test for tuberculosis.

Pharyngoscopy examination of the pharynx with a lighted instrument.

Pneumonectomy surgical removal of the lung.

Rhinoplasty reshaping the nose.

Rhinoscopy examination of the nose with a lighted instrument.

Spirogram measurement of respiratory movements with a special machine - spirograph.

Tine test skin test for tuberculosis.

Tracheostomy making an artificial opening into the trachea (allowing air to enter the bronchi and lungs to relieve obstruction to breathing).

Tracheotomy cutting into the trachea.

Underwater seal drainage the removal of air from the chest (thoracic) cavity by the insertion of a tube placed under water in a special drainage bottle.

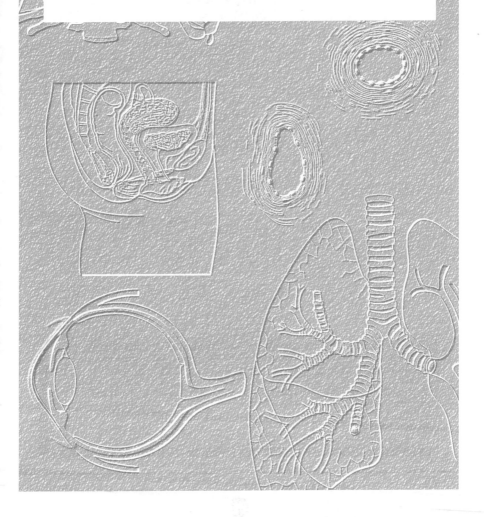

FUNCTION

This system is concerned with the intake, breakdown and absorption of food substances for use and storage by the body cells.

Food is taken into the mouth, chewed, mixed with saliva and formed into a **bolus** which, on swallowing, is passed into the **oesophagus**. From here it travels through the remainder of the alimentary canal by means of **peristalsis** (alternate waves of contraction and relaxation of

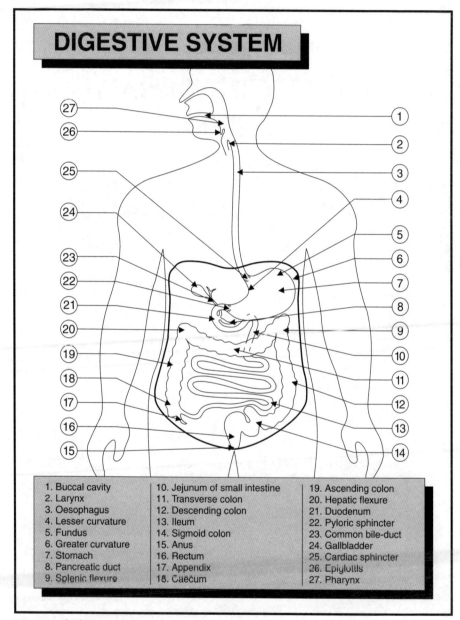

DIGESTIVE SYSTEM

1. Buccal cavity	10. Jejunum of small intestine	19. Ascending colon
2. Larynx	11. Transverse colon	20. Hepatic flexure
3. Oesophagus	12. Descending colon	21. Duodenum
4. Lesser curvature	13. Ileum	22. Pyloric sphincter
5. Fundus	14. Sigmoid colon	23. Common bile-duct
6. Greater curvature	15. Anus	24. Gallbladder
7. Stomach	16. Rectum	25. Cardiac sphincter
8. Pancreatic duct	17. Appendix	26. Epiglottis
9. Splenic flexure	18. Caecum	27. Pharynx

Figure 30 - The digestive system.

the muscular walls of the hollow organs). It mixes with the various digestive juices, secreted from glands situated in the lining of the stomach and small intestine. These juices contain enzymes which allow the chemical process of digestion to occur. Other substances are also received into the small intestine for this purpose, from the liver and pancreas, via ducts.

Digestion

This is both:

| physical | by means of chewing (mastication), peristalsis and churning (by muscular action of the stomach and intestinal walls) which reduce the food to smaller particles. |
| chemical | by the presence of chemicals, including substances known as **enzymes**. These allow chemical changes to occur enabling more simple compounds to be absorbed through the lining of the organs, especially in the **ileum** of the small intestine where most food substances are absorbed. |

STRUCTURE

The following organs form the system and are known as the **alimentary canal** (see Figure 30):

- mouth or **buccal cavity**
- **oral pharynx** (throat)
- **oesophagus** (gullet)
- **stomach**
- small intestine:
  - **duodenum**
  - **jejunum**
  - **ileum**
- large intestine:
  - **caecum**
  - **appendix**
  - **ascending colon**
  - **transverse colon**
  - **sigmoid colon**
  - **rectum**
  - **anus**

Oesophagus

This is a strong muscular tube, situated in the thoracic cavity, extending from the pharynx above to the stomach below. It penetrates the diaphragm at its junction with the stomach.

Stomach

This is the most dilated part of the alimentary canal, containing numerous glands, secreting enzymes and also mucus to protect its own tissues from digestion.

Gastric juice is produced, which includes enzymes, starting the digestion of protein, and hydrochloric acid aiding digestion. Absence of hydrochloric acid is common in **pernicious anaemia**.

It is guarded at the junction to the oesophagus by a weak sphincter muscle (**cardiac sphincter**). At its junction with the duodenum is a stronger sphincter known as the **pyloric sphincter**. These regulate the entrance and exit of, the now liquid, food substances known as **chyme**.

Sphincter muscles

A sphincter muscle consists of a ring of circular muscle which guards the entrance or exit of certain structures of the body. By its contraction or relaxation it controls the passage of various substances.

Small intestine

This consists of the **duodenum, jejunum** and **ileum**, each of which contributes to the mechanical and chemical digestion of food substances.

Numerous tiny projection-type structures, known as **villi**, are found in the lining of the small intestine, the most numerous being found in the ileum. It is through these specialised structures that most of the food substances reach the blood stream and fats, as fatty acids (**lipids**), are absorbed directly into the **lymphatic system** as chyle.

Ileocaecal reflex

Whenever food or liquid is swallowed and passes into the stomach, a reflex action occurs known as the ileocaecal reflex. This involves the passing of the liquid food substances from the last part of the ileum of the small intestine, into the **caecum** through the **ileocaecal valve**, a one-way valve.

Large intestine

This is also known as the **colon**. It consists of a long muscular tube, starting at the caecum, to which the **appendix** is attached, extending to the **anus** below. It is concerned with the reabsorption of water, mineral salts and vitamins, and the breakdown of indigestible matter (cellulose from plants) into faeces. At the act of defecation this is eliminated from the body via the anus. The anus is guarded by a voluntary sphincter muscle.

Certain vitamins, e.g. **vitamin K**, are manufactured here by the action of bacteria, naturally present in the bowel. Treatment with extended courses of oral antibiotics interfere with this function.

ACCESSORY ORGANS OF DIGESTION

These consist of the following structures:

- **teeth**
- **tongue** } in the mouth
- **salivary glands**
- **pancreas**
- **liver** } in abdominal cavity
- **gallbladder**

Teeth

There are 32 **permanent teeth** and 20 primary or **deciduous teeth** which are replaced in childhood and adolescence by the permanent or **secondary teeth**.

Tongue

The tongue, also involved in speech and perception of taste (see Section 14), is concerned with formation of a **bolus** (a ball of food mixed with saliva), which is moved to the back of the pharynx and swallowed (**deglutition**), travelling into the oesophagus. Difficulty with swallowing is known as **dysphagia**.

Salivary glands

The salivary glands secrete **saliva** which starts the digestion of cooked starches.

Pancreas

The pancreas is a gland producing **insulin**. It secretes **pancreatic juice** containing several enzymes which are carried via ducts to the duodenum where it aids in the digestion of proteins, starches and sugars.

Liver

The liver secretes bile which emulsifies fat ready for digestion and absorption. There are many other functions of the liver, including:

- The removal of nitrogen from proteins which are to be eliminated from the body (**deamination**).

- The breakdown of drugs and poisons ready for excretion by the kidneys (**detoxification**).

- Production of numerous enzymes.

- Production of clotting factors, including **prothrombin**, **fibrinogen** and anti-clotting factor **heparin**.

- Storage of essential vitamins, including **vitamins A, B, D and K**.

- Storage of **iron** from worn out blood cells, and the conversion of pigments into bile pigments (**bilirubin**) which colour the faeces in which they are excreted.

- Breakdown of many fatty acids (**desaturation**) ready for storage or use by the body.

- Conversion and storage of glucose ready for release into the blood stream.

- Production of heat for distribution via the blood stream to the rest of the body - the numerous chemical reactions occurring in the body produce heat.

Gallbladder

The gallbladder is an elongated sac located below the liver. It stores and concentrates bile which it receives from the liver via ducts, ready for release into the duodenum of the small intestine to mix with other enzymes secreted by the intestinal walls.

ABBREVIATIONS

ABC	aspiration, biopsy, cytology
abdo	abdomen/abdominal
Ba E	barium enema
Ba M	barium meal
BM	bowel movement
BO	bowels open
D&V	diarrhoea and vomiting
DU	duodenal ulcer
ERCP	endoscopic retrograde cholangiopancreatography
GI	gastrointestinal
GU	gastric ulcer
HCl	hydrochloric acid
Hp	*helicobacter pylori* (bacteria responsible for gastric ulcers)
IBS	irritable bowel syndrome
IUC	idiopathic ulcerative colitis

IVC	intravenous cholangiography
LIF	left iliac fossa
LIH	left inguinal hernia
LLQ	left lower quadrant
LUQ	left upper quadrant
OGD	oesophagogastroduodenoscopy
N&V	nausea and vomiting
NG	new growth/ nasogastric (tube)
PR	per rectum
PU	peptic ulcer
RIF	right/left iliac fossa
RIH	right/left inguinal hernia
RLQ	right lower quadrant
RUQ	right upper quadrant
UC	ulcerative colitis
UGI	upper gastrointestinal

TERMINOLOGY

An/o	stem for anus.
Appendic/o	stem for appendix.
Caec/o	stem for caecum.
Cholecyst/o	stem for gallbladder.
Choledoch/o	stem for common bile duct.
Col/o	stem for colon (large intestine).
Dent/o	tooth.
Duoden/o	stem for duodenum.
Gastr/o	stem for stomach.
Gingiv/o	stem for gums.
Hepat/o	stem for liver.
Ile/o	stem for ileum (part of small intestine).
Jejun/o	stem for jejunum.
Odont/o	tooth.
Oesophag/o	stem for oesophagus.
Pancreat/o	stem for pancreas.
Phag/o	swallow/eat.
Proct/o	rectum.
Pylor/o	part of stomach (pylorus).
Rect/o (proct/o)	stem for rectum.
Sigmoid/o	stem for sigmoid colon.
Stomat/o	stem for mouth.
Atresia	without a natural opening.
Biliary	concerning bile.
Caries	dental disease.
Deciduous teeth	primary/first teeth (20).

Orthodontal	concerned with the correction of dentition (teeth).
Orthodontist	specialists in correction of teeth.
Permanent teeth	secondary teeth (32).

DISEASES AND DISORDERS

Achlorhydria	absence of hydrochloric acid secretion in the stomach.
Acholia	absence of bile.
Adhesions	fibrous tissue formation causes abnormal joining of two organ surfaces.
Anal fissure	painful crack in the mucous membrane of the anus.
Anorexia	loss of appetite.
Anorexia nervosa	loss of appetite due to emotional states.
Appendicitis	inflammation of the appendix of the intestine.
Ascites	free fluid in the peritoneal cavity.
Barium enema	X-ray where barium compound (opaque medium) is inserted into the bowel via the rectum for diagnostic purposes.
Barium meal	as above, but taken by mouth.
Barium swallow	as above, but the swallowing process is also screened.
Cholecystitis	inflammation of the gallbladder.
Choledocholithiasis	condition of stones in the bile duct.
Cholelithiasis	condition of stones in the gallbladder.
Cirrhosis	hardening of an organ, usually the liver.
Coeliac disease	disease in which the protein gluten is not properly broken down - characterised by fatty stools (steatorrhoea) and failure to gain weight when it occurs in early childhood.

Colic	spasmodic waves of pain due to contraction of muscles in tubular organs.
Colitis	inflammation of the colon.
Crohn's disease	chronic inflammation of the last part of the ileum (small intestine).
Diverticulitis	inflammation of a pouch formation in the lining of the intestine.
Diverticulum	an abnormal pouch formation in the lining of a hollow organ, e.g. intestine.
Faecal vomiting	present when all bowel movements have ceased - obstruction, paralytic ileus - vomit consists of liquid faeces.
Fistula	abnormal communication between two organs or an organ with the skin.
Gastritis	inflammation of the stomach.
Gastroenteritis	inflammation of the stomach and intestine.
Gingivitis	inflammation of the gums.
Haematemesis	vomiting of blood from the stomach.
Haemorrhoidectomy	surgical removal of haemorrhoids.
Haemorrhoids	varicose veins of the rectum ('piles').
Helicobacter pylori	bacteria which live and reproduce in the gastric secretions of the stomach and may cause gastric ulcers.
Helminthiasis	infestation with intestinal worms.
Hepatitis	inflammation of the liver.
Hepatoma	malignant tumour of the liver.
Hepatomegaly	enlargement of the liver.
Hernia	abnormal protrusion of an organ or structure through a weakness in a muscle.
Hiatus hernia	protrusion of the stomach wall through a weakness in the diaphragm - allows regurgitation of acid contents.
Intestinal obstruction	an acute abdominal emergency - contents of intestine are unable to pass along due to obstruction, e.g. strangulated hernia.
Intussusception	the pushing of one part of the intestine into the lumen (space) of another part immediately adjacent to it; causes obstruction - common in children - an acute abdominal emergency.
Malocclusion	badly aligned teeth when closing mouth.
Melaena	black, tarry stools due to presence of digested blood (bleeding occurring).
Malnutrition	deficiency of quantity or quality of food eaten.
McBurney's point	area on the abdominal wall in the right iliac fossa where pain is felt when pressure is applied when diagnosing appendicitis.
Occult blood	hidden blood, not visible to the naked eye (in stools).
Oesophagitis	inflammation of the oesophagus (gullet).
Paralytic ileus	no bowel sounds heard with stethoscope indicating no movement (peristalsis).
Periodontal	area around the tooth.
Peritonitis	inflammation of the peritoneum (the membrane covering and nourishing the abdominal organs).

Pilonidal sinus	an abnormality consisting of an infolding of skin containing hair over the coccygeal area which has formed a space (sinus) and can become infected.
Plaque	tartar upon the teeth causing caries etc.
Proctalgia	pain in the rectum.
Pyloric stenosis	narrowing of the pyloric sphincter of the stomach (muscle fibres fail to relax sufficiently to allow passage of food from stomach into duodenum) - causes projectile vomiting, common in first-born male babies.
Pyorrhoea	discharge of pus from the tooth cavity.
Steatorrhoea	abnormal fatty stools.
Stomatitis	inflammation of the mouth.
Strangulated hernia	an acute abdominal emergency in which a portion of the alimentary canal protrudes through the muscle and becomes constricted, losing its blood supply - without intervention, gangrene will occur.
Ulcerative colitis	chronic inflammatory disease of the colon which causes diarrhoea, blood and mucus in the stools.
Volvulus	twisting of intestine upon itself, causing obstruction.

PROCEDURES AND EQUIPMENT

Abdominoperineal excision	surgical removal of rectum and part of colon and a colostomy created.
Anastomosis	surgical joining of two hollow organs.
Appendicectomy	surgical removal of the appendix.
Cholecystectomy	surgical removal of the gallbladder.
Colectomy	surgical removal of all or part of the colon.
Colostomy	making an artificial opening of the colon onto the abdominal wall.
Endoscopic retrograde cholangio-pancreatogram	special X-ray of gallbladder and pancreas using fluorescent dye which is inserted into ampulla of Vater ducts from duodenum using a duodenoscope with a catheter attached. It allows investigation of bile and pancreatic ducts and their contents. Cytology and biochemistry tests are performed.
Endoscopy	examination of a hollow organ with a lighted flexible tube - fibre optics.
Extraction	removal of (e.g.tooth).
Gastrectomy	surgical removal of the stomach.
Gastrojejunostomy	anastomosis (joining together) the stomach and jejunum having removed or bypassed the duodenum; **similar anastomosis terms follow this form**.
Gastroscope	lighted instrument used to examine the stomach.
Gastroscopy	examination of the stomach with a lighted instrument.
Gastrostomy	an artificial opening into the stomach, usually for feeding purposes.
Gastrotomy	cutting into the stomach.
Herniorrhaphy	surgical repair of a hernia.

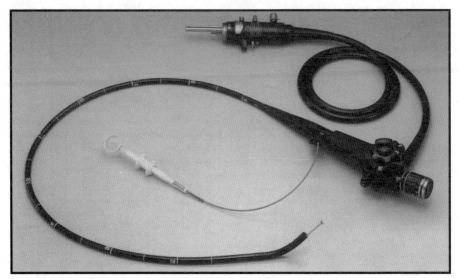

Figure 31 - A gastrointestinal fibrescope. Reproduced with kind permission from Keymed (Medical and Industrial Equipment) Ltd.

Ileostomy	making an artificial opening of the ileum onto the abdominal wall.	**Proctoscope**	lighted instrument for examination of the rectum.
Laparoscopy	examination of the abdomen with a lighted instrument through the abdominal wall.	**Proctoscopy**	examination of the rectum with a lighted instrument.
Laparotomy	incision into the abdominal wall for exploratory purposes.	**Ramstedt's operation**	cutting into tight muscle fibres of pyloric sphincter of stomach and reshaping the stomach wall (for pyloric stenosis in babies).
Oesophagectomy	surgical removal of the oesophagus.		

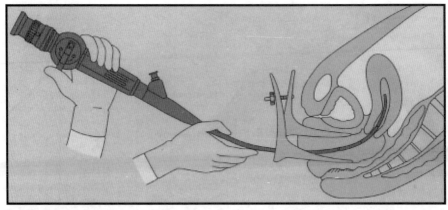

Figure 32 - Hysteroscopy. Reproduced with kind permission from Keymed (Medical and Industrial Equipment) Ltd.

Table 3 – Examples of endoscopies

Procedure	Examination	Description
Oesophagoscopy	oesophagus	use of oesophagoscope for visual examination of oesophagus or removal of foreign body
Gastroscopy	stomach	visual examination of stomach using a gastroscope inserted via the mouth and oesophagus. Biopsy and aspiration are performed
Duodenoscopy	duodenum (part of small intestine)	visual examination of duodenum via mouth, oesophagus and stomach. Biopsy and aspiration are performed
Colonoscopy	large intestine	visual examination of colon via rectum using a colonoscope. Polyps may be removed and a biopsy performed
Sigmoidoscopy	sigmoid area of large intestine	visual examination of the sigmoid colon via the rectum using a sigmoidoscope. Polyps may be removed and a biopsy performed
Proctosigmoidoscopy	rectum and sigmoid area	visual examination using proctoscope or sigmoidoscope. Polyps may be removed and a biopsy performed
Endoscopic retrograde cholangiopancreatography	bile and pancreatic ducts	X-ray by insertion of dye into ampulla of Vater via catheter attached to endoscope inserted into duodenum

ENDOSCOPY

Endoscopy is the examination of a canal or hollow organ with a lighted instrument (Figures 31 and 32). The conventional endoscope is rigid and non-flexible which has been widely replaced by the flexible fibre-optic variety. The endoscope is inserted into a hollow organ or tube such as the alimentary canal. Visual examination is performed and photography, biopsy and aspiration are carried out in appropriate cases (Table 3).

Commonly, an oesophagogastroduodenoscopy (OGD) is performed which examines all three areas of the alimentary canal. Any lesion or abnormality can be seen and samples can be taken for histology.

OTHER COMMON ENDOSCOPIES

Procedure	Examination of
Laryngoscopy	larynx (voice box)
Tracheoscopy	trachea (windpipe)
Bronchoscopy	bronchial tubes
Laparoscopy	lower abdominal cavity via the umbilicus

	(also used for biopsy of ovaries and female sterilisation)	**Hysteroscopy**	cavity of uterus
		Cystoscopy	bladder
		Retinoscopy	retina of eye
Colposcopy	vagina	**Rhinoscopy**	nasal cavities
Culdoscopy	through the recto-uterine pouch of pelvic peritoneum (pouch of Douglas) to view pelvic cavity	**Otoscopy**	ear canal

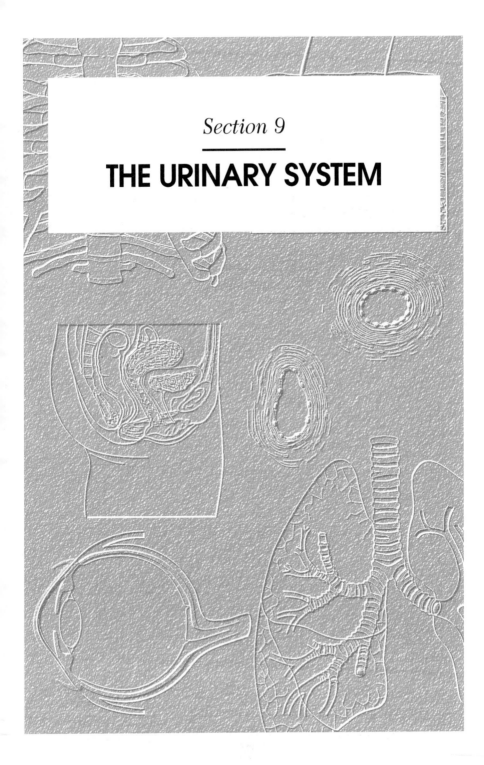

Section 9

THE URINARY SYSTEM

The urinary system is concerned with the removal of waste products from the body and the maintenance of correct water and **electrolyte** (ion) levels.

FUNCTION

The kidneys remove the nitrogenous content from the protein food substances which have not been utilised by the body, after they have been broken down for excretion by the liver (deamination). Protein cannot be stored by the body. Drugs and toxins are also removed in this way.

The kidneys act as filters and also selectively secrete and reabsorb substances from the blood to maintain the correct balance of salts, water and other substances. This is an example of **homeostasis**, whereby the body is kept in the correct state for functioning. A sufficiently high blood pressure is necessary for this to occur and any prolonged condition of extreme **hypotension** (abnormally low blood pressure) can cause permanent damage to the kidneys.

STRUCTURE

It comprises the following organs (see Figure 33):

- Two **kidneys**
- Two **ureters**
- **Bladder**
- **Urethra**

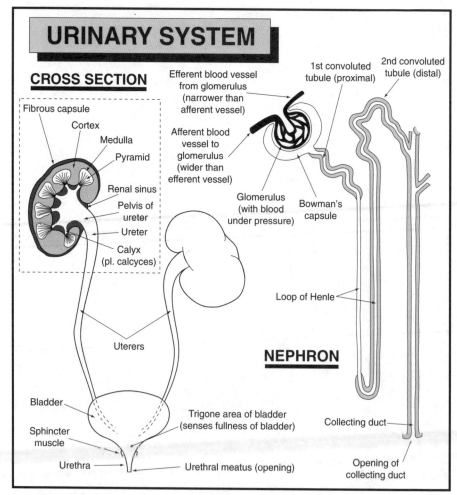

Figure 33 - *The urinary system.*

Kidneys

Kidneys are brown/purple bean-shaped vascular organs which are divided into lobules. They lie on the posterior part of the abdominal cavity deeply embedded in fat, and are surrounded by a capsule consisting of an outer portion, the **cortex**, and an inner portion, the **medulla**. The medulla shows striations called pyramids; these project into the pelvis of the kidney which is continuous with the ureter. On the upper pole of each kidney is the **adrenal** or **supra-renal** gland.

Microscopic structure of kidneys

The complex structures forming the kidneys are called **nephrons**, of which there are approximately 1 million in each. A nephron consists of a structure called a **Malpighian body** (in which filtration occurs) and various tubules, where substances are either secreted from or reabsorbed into the blood. Nephrons have a very rich blood supply.

Nephron

The nephron consists of the following microscopic structures:
- **Glomerulus**, collectively known as Malpighian body or **glomeruli** apparatus
- **Bowman's** capsule
- **First convoluted tubule (proximal)**
- **Loop of Henle**
- **Second convoluted tubule (distal)**
- **Collecting tubule**

Malpighian body or glomeruli apparatus

A Malpighian body, also known as the glomeruli apparatus, consists of the glomerulus and a cup-shaped tubular structure called the Bowman's capsule. The glomerulus consists of a tuft of capillaries tightly packed into the Bowman's capsule, which is the expanded commencement of a 'uriniferous' or kidney tubule.

The small arteries leading into the glomerulus (afferent vessels) are wider than the arteries leaving the glomerulus (efferent vessels), thus back-pressure arises to allow **filtration** of substances from the blood to occur in the Bowman's capsule.

Tubules

The first convoluted tubule (proximal tubule) is coiled and continuous with the Bowman's capsule, the loop of Henle which dips down into the medulla of the kidney, and the second convoluted tubule (distal tubule) which joins the collecting tubule, also situated in the medulla. The collecting tubule terminates at a cup-shaped structure called the **calyx** (plural calyces) which opens into the pelvis of the kidney.

The Malpighian bodies and convoluted tubules are found in the cortex of the kidney where they are richly supplied with blood.

Formation of urine

Urine is formed by the following processes:
- **Filtration** – Non-selective
- **Secretion** – Selective
- **Reabsorption**

Filtration

Filtration is a non-selective process which takes place in the Malpighian bodies. Water, salts, glucose, urea, uric acid and toxins are filtered from the blood in the glomerulus into the Bowman's capsule (pressure in the glomerulus is high due to the efferent arteries being narrower than the afferent vessels). The capillary walls are more permeable than those elsewhere in the body. The fluid produced in the Bowman's capsule by this pressure is known as **filtrate**.

Secretion

Secretion occurs mainly in the first and second convoluted tubules. Special secretory cells line the tubules and **selectively** secrete substances from the blood which are at a high level, e.g. glucose in cases of diabetes mellitus. Foreign substances such as drugs and toxins will also be secreted. Similarly, any waste products of metabolism which have not already been filtered will be secreted into the tubules.

Reabsorption

Harm would occur if all the fluid, salts and food substances (such as glucose) filtered from the blood were allowed to leave the body. Specialised cells **selectively** reabsorb the necessary factors. In the loop of Henle most of the water is reabsorbed and the salt balance is restored mainly in the second convoluted tubule. The **'renal threshold'** (whereby the level of various substances retained or excreted by the kidneys is governed by the requirements of the body) is another example of homeostasis.

Hormones influence reabsorption; **aldosterone** secreted by the adrenal cortex stimulates the sodium/potassium reabsorption or secretion by the second convoluted tubule. The action of the pituitary hormone, **anti-diuretic hormone (ADH)**, influences the amount of water reabsorbed.

After all these processes the end product is urine which is acid in reaction. This passes to the collecting tubules and then into the pelvis of the kidney. Approximately 1 litre of urine is secreted in 24 hours.

Kidney damage

Any damage or disease to the kidney will obviously affect the processes of filtration, secretion and reabsorption, resulting in many beneficial factors, such as the protein albumin being lost from the body. Not all harmful substances and waste products will be excreted. If the damage is sufficient, then the resultant renal failure may require **dialysis** (the removal of waste products by artificial means) or a kidney transplant.

Erythropoietin and renin

The kidneys also secrete a hormone known as erythropoietin which affects the production of red blood cells. In patients on permanent dialysis these red blood cells can become depleted, causing anaemia. The hormone renin is also produced by the kidneys and helps to maintain blood pressure. It acts by converting one of the blood proteins into **angiotensin** which causes constriction of the arterioles, thus raising blood pressure.

Pelvis of the kidney

The dilated portion of the kidney, which acts as a funnel for the collection of the secreted urine from the tubules, is known as the **pelvis of the kidney**. Urine passes through this on its way to the ureters.

Ureters

These are two muscular tubes which convey urine from the kidneys to the bladder. They are joined obliquely to the base of the bladder at an area known as the **trigone**.

Bladder

This is a hollow, pear-shaped muscular sac where urine is stored before **micturition** (passing of urine) through the urethral **meatus** (opening). It is capable of great expansion and rises in the abdomen as it fills. Micturition is a reflex action which, after infancy, is normally controlled at will. In **incontinence** this property is lost.

Normal content of the bladder is approximately 150 ml, but it can hold up to 350-400 ml. A **sphincter muscle** guards the bladder opening.

Urethra

This is a muscular tube through which the urine is passed to the outside of the body. It is short in the female - one to two inches in length - and seven to eight inches in the male. It is guarded by a **sphincter muscle**.

COMPOSITION OF URINE

Normal urine has the following composition: straw-coloured acid fluid pH 5-7, containing -

Water	96%
Solids	2% salts
Nitrogenous products	
of urea and uric acid	2%
Creatinine – waste product	
of cell metabolism	

ABBREVIATIONS

AGN	acute glomeru-lonephritis
BNO	bladder neck obstruction
CAPD	continuous ambulatory peritoneal dialysis
C&S	culture and sensitivity (to grow any micro-organisms and determine the antibiotic to which they are sensitive)
CSU	catheter specimen of urine
EMU	early morning urine
ESL	extracorporeal shock-wave lithotripsy
GU	genitourinary
HPU	has passed urine
HNPU	has not passed urine
KUB	kidney, ureter, and bladder (X-ray)
MSU	midstream specimen of urine
NAD	no abnormality detected/demonstrated
NOAD	no other abnormality demonstrated
IVP	intravenous pyelogram
IVU	intravenous urogram
pH	acid/alkaline balance
RCP	retrograde pyelogram
UA	urinalysis
UTI	urinary tract infection
VCU	voiding cystourethrogram

| VCUG | voiding cystourethrogram |

TERMINOLOGY

Cyst/o	stem for bladder.
Glomerul/o	stem for glomerulus (part of nephron).
Nephr/o (pyel/o, ren/o)	stem for kidney.
Ur/o	stem for urine.
Ureter/o	stem for ureter.
Urethr/o	stem for urethra.
Urin/o	stem for urine.
-uria	suffix for condition of urine.
Genitourologist	specialist in the treatment of sexually transmitted diseases.
Glomerulus	small tuft of capillaries found within Bowman's capsule, forming part of the nephron.
Micturition	the act of passing urine.
Urologist	specialist in diseases of the urinary system.
Urology	study of the urinary system.

DISEASES AND DISORDERS

Albuminuria	the abnormal presence of albumin in the urine (protein).
Anuria	suppression of urine secretion from the kidneys - renal failure.
Bilirubinuria	presence of bile pigments in the urine.
Biluria	presence of bile salts in the urine.
Cystalgia	pain in the bladder.
Cystitis	inflammation of the bladder.
Cystocele	protrusion of the bladder, usually into the vaginal wall.
Cystolithiasis	condition of stones in the bladder.
Diuresis	increase in the production of urine.
Dysuria	difficulty/pain in passing urine.
Enuresis	bedwetting.
Glomerulonephritis	any of a group of kidney diseases involving the glomeruli.
Glycosuria	presence of glucose in the urine.
Haematuria	presence of blood in the urine.
Hydronephrosis	backlog of urine in the pelvis causing pressure and damaging the kidney.
Incontinence	inability to control the passing of urine or faeces.
Ketonuria	presence of acetone in the urine.
Nephritis	inflammation of the kidney.
Nephrolith	a kidney stone (calcium salts).
Nephrolithiasis	the condition of stones in the kidney.
Nephropathy	degenerative disease of the kidney.
Nephrosis	disease of the kidney.
Nephrotic syndrome	extensive signs and symptoms of kidney disease; can be caused by a variety of disorders, usually glomerulonephritis.
Nephrotomy	cutting into the kidney.
Nocturnal enuresis	bedwetting at night.
Oliguria	scanty production of urine.
Papilloma	a simple benign tumour of the bladder lining - can become malignant.
Phenylketonuria (PKU)	presence of abnormal breakdown of protein in urine in hereditary disease of PKU, screened for at birth as causes mental deficiency if not treated.
Polydipsia	excessive thirst.
Polyuria	passing large amounts of urine.
Pyelitis	inflammation of the pelvis of the kidney.
Pyelonephritis	inflammation of the kidney and its pelvis.
Pyuria	presence of pus in the urine.

Renal calculus	kidney stone.
Renal colic	severe spasmodic pain caused by presence of kidney stones in the renal system (kidneys or tubules).
Renal failure	the kidneys fail to produce sufficient urine to remove waste substances from the blood.
Urethral stricture	narrowing of the urethra.
Uraemia	high levels of urea (the waste part containing nitrogen) in the blood.
Ureteritis	inflammation of the ureters.
Ureterolith	stone in the ureter.
Ureterolithiasis	condition of stones in the ureters.
Urethritis	inflammation of the urethra.
Urethrocele	protrusion of the urethra, usually into the anterior vaginal wall.

PROCEDURES AND EQUIPMENT

Catheterisation	the withdrawal of urine from the bladder by the insertion of a catheter (fine hollow tube) into the urethra.
Continuous ambulant peritoneal dialysis (CAPD)	removing toxins and waste products from the body in kidney failure by passing the peritoneal fluid through a bag (containing chemicals) attached to the abdomen.
Cystectomy	surgical removal of the bladder.
Cystoscope	instrument used to examine the bladder.
Cystoscopy	examination of the bladder with a lighted instrument.

Dialysis	artificial filtration of the blood to remove waste products by machine or by chemical means (peritoneal dialysis).
Extracorporeal shock-wave lithotripsy	see lithotriptor.
Intravenous pyelogram	special X-ray demonstrating the shape and condition of the kidneys, ureters and bladder by intravenous injection of an opaque dye into the veins of the arm.
Lithotripsy	the breaking up of kidney stones (calculi) by a lithotriptor.
Lithotriptor	a machine which is used to break up stones by use of shock waves (pieces are then passed in the urine).
Micturating cystogram	special X-ray of the bladder when passing urine to demonstrate any weakness in muscles.
Micturition	act of passing urine.
Nephrectomy	surgical removal of the kidney.
Peritoneal dialysis	artificial removal of waste products from the blood by means of passing peritoneal fluid from the abdominal cavity through a chemical (externally).
Retrograde pyelogram	special X-ray of the kidney pelvis ureters and bladder by the insertion of fine catheters via the urethra and insertion of an opaque dye.
Ureterotomy	cutting into the ureter.
Voiding cystourethrogram	see micturating cystogram. Urethra is also demonstrated.

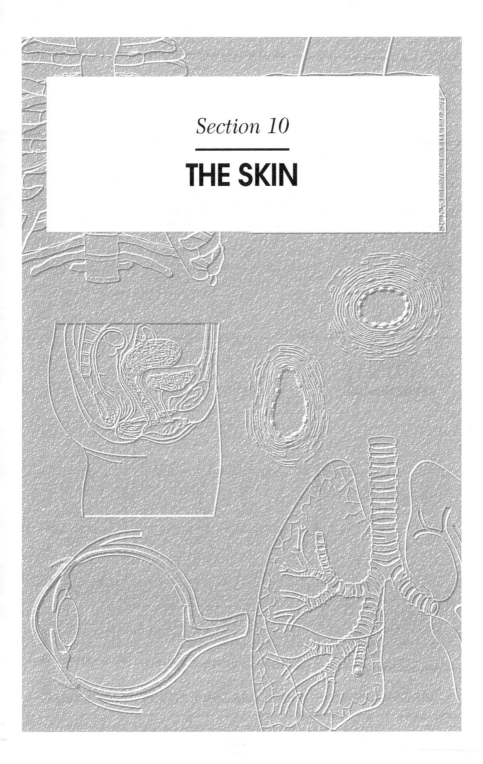

Section 10

THE SKIN

The skin is a vital organ which covers the whole of the body surface and is continuous with the **mucous membranes**.

STRUCTURE

It is composed of (see Figure 34):

- **Epidermis**
- **Dermis**
- Appendages of **hair** and **nails**

Epidermis

This is the uppermost layer of the skin and consists of several layers of epithelial-type cells. The top layers have no nucleus and are flattened and scaly. This is known as the horny layer or **keratin scales**. They are constantly being rubbed away and shed. These areas are thicker in various areas of the body which have to withstand friction and pressure, e.g. soles of feet.

The bottom layer of the epidermis, known as the **Basal (Malpighian) layer**, is the germinative layer from which these cells originate. It is here that the pigmentation (**melanin**), which gives rise to the colour of the skin, is found. There are no blood vessels in this layer and it is nourished by **lymph**.

Dermis

This is the layer found beneath the epidermis. It is composed of dense connective tissue containing elastic fibres and numerous structures:

- **blood vessels**
- **sensory nerve endings**
- **hair follicles** attached to small muscles
- **sweat glands**
- **sebaceous glands**

Blood vessels are numerous and are concerned not only with nourishment and delivery of vital substances to the skin, but also with the control of body temperature.

Sensory nerve endings are concerned with the relay of messages to the brain concerning touch, pressure, pain and temperature changes.

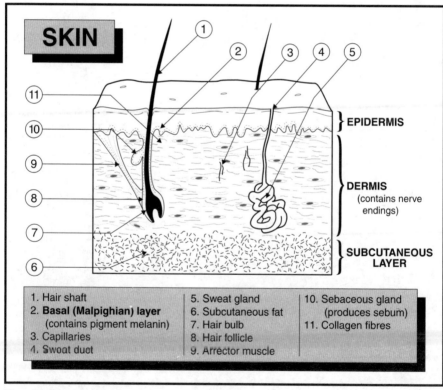

Figure 34 - Structure of the skin.

Sweat glands

These are concerned in the production of **sweat**, which excretes waste substances of water and salts from the body and also aids in the control of body temperature by loss of heat through **evaporation**.

Sebaceous glands

These produce a substance known as **sebum** which keeps the skin and hairs supple. Blockage of the duct of the gland produces a condition known as a **sebaceous cyst**.

Appendages

The hairs and nails are found in the dermis but are really outgrowths of the **epidermal layer**, as are sweat and sebaceous glands. Nails are protective and are outgrowths of the horny layer of the epidermis.

Beneath the dermis is a **subcutaneous layer** of connective tissue containing fat which helps to prevent heat loss.

FUNCTION

Control of body temperature

This is one of the main functions of the skin and is under the control of the brain. Special cells in the brain centre are triggered by the temperature of the blood flowing through it which, when the body temperature is becoming too hot, cause dilatation of the blood vessels in the skin, thus bringing more blood closer to the surface of the body. Sweat glands are stimulated to produce more sweat, excreting it through the pores onto the body surface where it evaporates. **Evaporation** is a very efficient form of heat loss. **Radiation, convection** and **conduction** from the body surface also contribute to loss of body heat.

Conversely, blood vessels constrict causing a transfer of blood to the centre of the body (**core**) and less heat is lost. Small muscles attached to hairs make them erect and cause 'goose pimples' which are an attempt to produce heat and allow hairs to trap air to provide insulation of the body, when it is cold. This is a remaining reflex from a more primitive form of life in evolution, when the body was covered in hair.

The average body temperature is 37°C, but varies during the day being lower in the morning.

Summary of other functions

- **Protection** by preventing micro-organisms entering the body and causing infection.
- **Preservation of** body fluid.
- **Conveys sensations** of touch, temperature, pain and pressure to the brain.
- **Produces sweat** and excretes waste products by this action.
- **Produces sebum**.
- Converts a substance known as **ergosterol**, present in skin, to **vitamin D** in the presence of ultraviolet light in sunshine. This vitamin is necessary for healthy bones and teeth.
- It is capable of **absorbing** some drugs, e.g. anti-inflammatory drugs.
- It gives origin to the **hair** and **nails** which continue to grow for a short time after death.

ABBREVIATIONS

DLE	disseminated lupus erythematosus
SLE	systemic lupus erythematosus

TERMINOLOGY

Derma/to	stem for skin.
Cutane/o	skin.
Hidr/o	sweat.
Onych/o	stem for nail.
Pil/o	hair.
Trich/o	stem for hair.
Ungu/o	nails.
Dermatologist	medical specialist of skin diseases.
Percutaneous	through the skin (infusions).
Subcutaneous	under the dermis layer of the skin.

DISEASES AND DISORDERS
(see Figure 35)

Abscess	collection of pus in a cavity.
Acne rosacea	skin disease due to thinning of the skin producing acne-like spots - can be caused by excessive use of steroid skin applications.
Acne vulgaris	skin disease - inflammation of sebaceous glands causing papules (red spots) and pustules to

form - common in adolescence.

Bullae	large (fluid containing) blisters.
Cellulitis	inflammation of the subcutaneous layer of the skin.
Chancre	an ulcer-type sore - primary stage of syphilis.
Comedone	blackhead.
Contusion	bruise - bleeding beneath the skin.
Cyst	membrane - encapsulated sac containing fluid or other materials.
Decubitus ulcer	bed sore (pressure sore).
Dermatitis	inflammation of the skin.
Dermatosis	disease of the skin.
Dermoid cyst	cyst present at birth containing embryonic materials - skin, nails, teeth etc. Usually found in the ovary.
Eczema	inflammatory skin disease due to allergy, usually against food, common in flexures of skin.
Erosion	rubbing away of tissues.
Erysipelas	acute contagious condition of the skin causing pain, fever and local inflammation of skin, usually on the face (caused by haemolytic streptococcus bacteria).
Erythema	reddening of skin.
Excoriation	injury worsened by act of friction (scratching).
Exfoliation	scaling of skin tissue in layers.
Fissure	a split or cleft.
Folliculitis	inflammation of a hair follicle.
Furuncle	a boil - an infection of the tissue around a hair follicle.
Haemangioma	birth mark (e.g. port wine type).
Herpes simplex	virus causing skin infection, usually cold sores.
Herpes zoster	painful shingles skin eruption along nerve path due to chicken pox virus.
Hidrosis	sweating.
Hirsuitism	excessive amount of body hair.
Hives	(also known as urticaria) weal-type spots due to allergy, as in nettle rash.
Hyperhidrosis	excessive production of sweat.
Impetigo	acute contagious disease producing pustules and scabs.
Keloid scar	overgrowth of scar tissue.
Lesion	any abnormal change in tissue.
Lupus erythematosus	inflammatory dermatitis characterised by 'butterfly' lesion over nose and cheeks; may become widespread and destroy vital tissues.
Macula	spot or discolouration of skin not raised above the surface, e.g. measles rash.
Malignant melanoma	virulent cancerous invasive type of melanin- (pigment-) producing cells.
Melanoma	pigmented mole of melanin-producing cells.
Morbilliform	describing a type of rash - similar to measles rash.
Naevus	birth mark.
Nodule	a small node (protuberence or swelling).
Onychogryphosis	thickened deformed nails.
Pachydermatous	thickened skin.
Papilloma	simple tumour (not malignant).
Papule	spot - small raised solid elevation.
Paronychia	infection of a nailbed

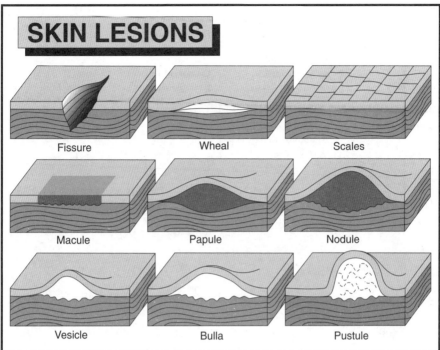

SKIN LESIONS

Fissure

Wheal

Scales

Macule

Papule

Nodule

Vesicle

Bulla

Pustule

Figure 35 - Skin lesions. Redrawn after Glylys BA (1995) Medical Terminology: A Systems Approach, 3rd edn. FA Davis.

Paronychia	infection of a nailbed (whitlow).		as in secondary syphilis.
Pediculosis	infestation with lice.	**Scabies**	infestation with the parasite scabies mite producing itching and soreness.
Pemphigus	blister-like eruptions which can be acute or chronic.		
Petechiae	small purplish patches under skin due to fluid escaped from small blood vessels - can be sign of recent asphyxiation or pressure.	**Scales**	compact layers of epithelial tissue shed from the skin.
		Seborrhoea	overactivity of the sebaceous glands which produce excessive sebum.
Prodromal rash	a fleeting rash which appears before the true rash of an infectious disease.	**Tinea pedis**	athlete's foot.
		Trichosis	any abnormal state of hair.
Pruritus	irritation of the skin.	**Ulcer**	an open sore of skin or mucous membranes.
Psoriasis	chronic skin disease characterised by scaly patches of unknown cause.	**Urticaria**	nettle rash, an allergic reaction.
		Vesicle	small fluid-filled blister.
Pustule	pus-filled small elevation of the skin.	**Vitiligo**	patchy white depigmentation of the skin.
Roseola	a rose-coloured rash		

Wart (verucca)   an epidermal tumour of viral origin, or any benign hardening.

Wheal   an acute reaction of the skin in nettle rash/urticaria/hives.

Xeroderma   abnormally dry skin.

PROCEDURES AND EQUIPMENT

Débridement   surgical cleaning of wounds by removing dead tissues.

Dermatology   scientific study of the skin.

Dermatome   instrument used to cut very thin layers of skin for skin grafting.

Escharectomy   removal of scar tissue.

Escharotomy   dividing burn-scar tissue (to prevent scarring).

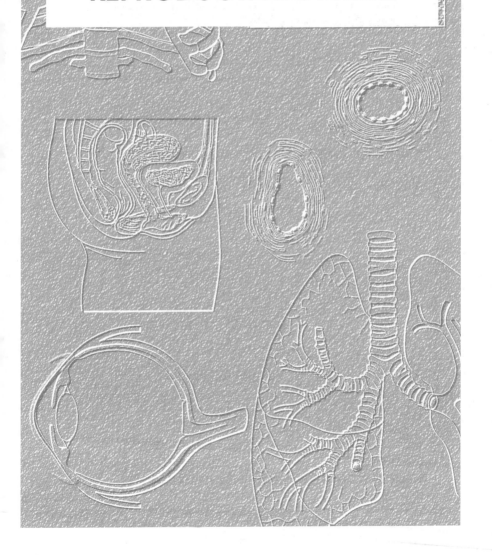

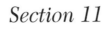
THE FEMALE REPRODUCTIVE SYSTEM

This system is concerned in the **reproduction** of the species (see Figures 36 and 37).

STRUCTURE

It is composed of both internal and external organs:

Internal organs

- Two **ovaries**
- Two **fallopian** tubes
- **Uterus**
- **Vagina**

} situated in the pelvic cavity

Ovaries

The ovaries, situated in the pelvic cavity, are the female **gonads** and produce **ova** (eggs) after menstruation starts (**menarche**). They are under the influence of the hormones from the **pituitary gland** and produce the female sex hormones **oestrogen** and **progesterone** at different stages of the menstrual cycle. Oestrogen is responsible for the development of the female sexual characteristics, while **progesterone**, produced in the second phase of the menstrual cycle, supplements the action of oestrogen by thickening the lining of the uterus ready for the possible implantation of a fertilised egg. It also stimulates the breasts, preparing them for **lactation**. The female is born with all the eggs (immature) present at birth. Normally only one egg (**ovum**) ripens and is released each month.

At the menopause (**climacteric**), egg production and hormonal secretion cease, although the adrenal gland cortex continues to influence the production of sex hormones at a lower level.

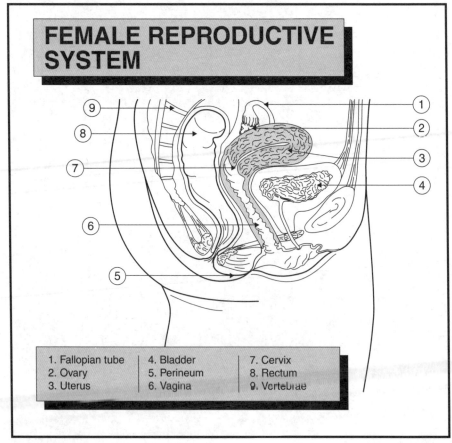

FEMALE REPRODUCTIVE SYSTEM

1. Fallopian tube	4. Bladder	7. Cervix
2. Ovary	5. Perineum	8. Rectum
3. Uterus	6. Vagina	9. Vertebrae

Figure 36 - Female reproductive system (side view).

Fallopian tubes

These are situated one each side of the uterus, and attached to the ovaries by fine, finger-like strands. They are composed of muscle and are hollow tube-like structures which carry the released ovum along into the uterus ready for embedding, or shedding if fertilisation has not occurred. **Fertilisation** occurs when the male spermatazoon fuses with the ovum in the fallopian tube.

Uterus

This consists of a muscular pear-shaped hollow organ partially covered in a layer of membrane known as the **peritoneum**. It normally slopes forwards (anteverted).

The three layers are the:

- **peritoneum**
- **myometrium**
- **endometrium**

The neck of the uterus is known as the **cervix** and protrudes into the vagina which envelopes it.

The **endometrium**, the lining of the uterus, is under the influence of the female hormones and is the site for the embedding of the fertilised ovum. If fertilisation and embedding do not occur, the lining is shed in monthly menstruation.

Vagina

This is a muscular tube-like structure of vascular, erectile tissue extending from the **cervix** of the uterus above to the **vulva** externally below. Its function is for the deposit of the male spermatazoa, a passage way for menstruation and the birth of a baby. Its walls are convoluted to allow for expansion.

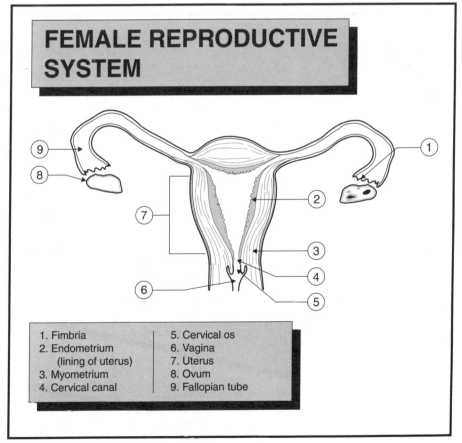

FEMALE REPRODUCTIVE SYSTEM

1. Fimbria
2. Endometrium (lining of uterus)
3. Myometrium
4. Cervical canal
5. Cervical os
6. Vagina
7. Uterus
8. Ovum
9. Fallopian tube

Figure 37 - Female reproductive system (front view).

EXTERNAL GENITAL ORGANS

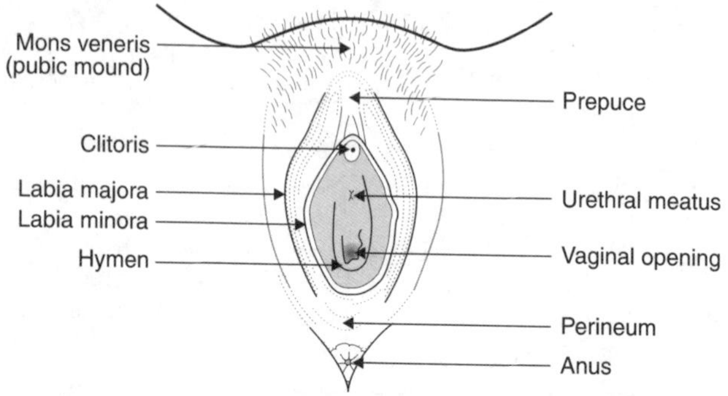

Mons veneris (pubic mound) — Prepuce
Clitoris
Labia majora — Urethral meatus
Labia minora
Hymen — Vaginal opening
— Perineum
— Anus

Figure 38 - The external organs.

External organs

Collectively these are known as the **vulva** (see Figure 38). They consist of the:

Bartholin's glands	two glands, one in each of the labia minora providing a secretion lubricating the vestibule.
Clitoris	a rudimentary penis of erectile tissue (becomes engorged with blood).
Hymen	thin membrane guarding the entrance to the vagina.
Labia majora	large outer lips.
Labia minora	smaller inner lips.
Mons veneris	pad of fat upon the pubis.
Perineum	area of skin and muscle extending from the vagina to the anus.
Vestibule	opening containing entrance to vagina and urethral meatus (opening).

THE BREASTS

The breasts, or **mammary glands**, are the accessory glands of the female reproductive system. They are rudimentary in the male. Their function is to produce milk for feeding the newborn baby.

Development

At puberty they enlarge and develop in the female, being under the influence of the female hormones. In pregnancy they increase in size and are stimulated ready to produce milk following delivery. They atrophy in old age.

Structure

The milk-secreting glands are found in **lobes** grouped together in **lobules**, separated by fibrous connective and fatty tissue. Each lobule opens into tubules, known as **lactiferous ducts**, which unite to form the main ducts terminating at the **nipple** (see Figure 39).

Hormone influence

The influence of the female hormones, **oestrogen** and **progesterone**, secreted by the ovaries at puberty and the start of menstruation, causes the enlargement and development of the breasts ready for future suckling.

In pregnancy, the production of progesterone by the **placenta** also influences further enlargement and development.

Prolactin (**LTH**), a hormone secretion of the anterior part of the **pituitary gland**, stimulates the production of milk. **Oxytocin**, from the pos-

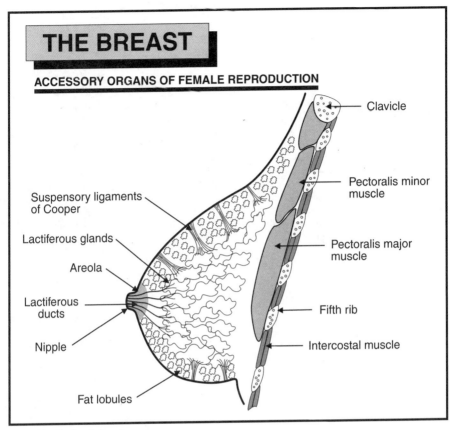

THE BREAST

ACCESSORY ORGANS OF FEMALE REPRODUCTION

- Clavicle
- Pectoralis minor muscle
- Pectoralis major muscle
- Fifth rib
- Intercostal muscle
- Suspensory ligaments of Cooper
- Lactiferous glands
- Areola
- Lactiferous ducts
- Nipple
- Fat lobules

Figure 39 - The female breast.

terior part of the pituitary gland, stimulates the **ejection** (or let down) of milk from the breast. **Suckling** encourages more milk to be produced.

Milk

This is a complete food for the newborn and is the most suitable nourishment for the human baby, having the correct proportions of nutrients. Cow's milk contains a larger proportion of protein which is not easily digestible, being very complex. Numerous **antibodies** produced by the mother are also present and help to prevent infection occurring in the baby.

Colostrum

During the latter part of pregnancy, a yellowish clear fluid, known as **colostrum**, containing sugar and protein, is produced. The milk production does not normally occur until the second or third

day following birth. This substance provides nourishment and also acts as an **aperient** to remove secretions present in the newborn's intestine.

ABBREVIATIONS

A&W	alive and well
ab	abortion
AFP	alphafetoprotein (test for abnormality in fetus) in amniotic fluid or maternal blood
AI	artificial insemination
AID	artificial insemination by donor
AIH	artificial insemination by husband
AN	antenatal
APH	antepartum

haemorrhage

ARM	artificial rupture of membranes
BBA	born before arrival
BSO	bilateral salpingo-oophorectomy (surgical removal of both fallopian tubes and both ovaries)
BW	birth weight
CIN	cervical intra-epithelial neoplasia (cervical pre-cancer). It is graded from one to three depending on degree of abnormality.
COC	combined oral contraceptive pill
CVS	chorionic villus sampling (to detect fetal abnomalities)
Cx	cervix (neck of womb)
D&C	dilatation and curettage (scraping out of womb)
DUB	dysfunctional uterine bleeding
EDC	expected date of confinement
EDD	expected date of delivery
EMU	early morning urine
ERPC	evacuation of retained products of conception
EUA	examination under anaesthetic
FHH	fetal heart heard
FHNH	fetal heart not heard
FMF	fetal movements felt
G&A	gas and air
HPL	human placental lactogen assay blood test (monitors health of placenta and fetus)
HRT	hormone replacement therapy
HSV	herpes simplex virus
HVS	high vaginal swab
IUCD	intra-uterine contraceptive device
IUD	intra-uterine device or intra-uterine death

IUFB	intra-uterine foreign body
IVF	*in vitro* fertilisation
LMP	last menstrual period

Positions of baby in utero:

LOA	left occipitoanterior (or ROA, right)
LOL	left occipitolateral
LOP	left occipitoposterior

LSCS	lower section caesarean section
NAI	non-accidental injury
ND	normal delivery
PAP	Papanicolaou smear (cervical smear test)
PCB	post-coital bleeding
PET	pre-eclamptic toxaemia
PID	pelvic inflammatory disease (also prolapsed intervertebral disc)
PMB	postmenopausal bleeding
PMS	premenstrual syndrome
PN	postnatal
PNC	postnatal clinic
POD	pouch of Douglas (fold of peritoneum lying behind the womb)
POP	progestogen only pill (contraceptive)
PP	placenta praevia
PPH	postpartum haemorrhage
PV	per vaginam
RDS	respiratory distress syndrome
RVS	respiratory virus syndrome
SB	still birth
SCAN	suspected child abuse or neglect
SCBU	special care baby unit
SI	sexual intercourse
SIDS	sudden infant death syndrome
STD	sexually transmitted disease
STYCAR	standard tests for young children and retardates, developed by Sheridan to assess visual development

TAH	total abdominal hysterectomy
TCRE	transcervical resection of endometrium
TOP	termination of pregnancy
TSS	toxic shock syndrome
TUP	tubal uterine pregnancy
TV	trichomonas vaginalis (infection of vagina causing frothy yellow discharge)
TVH	total vaginal hysterectomy
USS	ultrasound scan
VI	virgo intacto (virgin)
Vx	vertex (the crown of the head of the fetus)
XX	female sex chromosomes
XY	male sex chromosomes

TERMINOLOGY

colp/o	stem for vagina.
nat/o	stem for birth.
men/o	stem for period.
uter/o	stem for womb.
vagin/o	stem for vagina.
vulv/o	stem for vulva.
-gravida	suffix for pregnancy.
-para, -partum	suffix for having given birth.
-tocia	suffix for labour.
Mamm/o (mast/o)	stem for breast.
Gynaec/o	stem for female.
Hyster/o (metr/o)	stem for womb/uterus.
Oophor/o (ovari/o)	stem for ovary.
Salping/o	stem for fallopian tube.
Amniotic membrane	the innermost layer which encloses the fetus and produces amniotic fluid.
Antenatal care	care given to both mother and fetus during pregnancy.
Anteverted uterus	normal forward tilting of the womb.
Braxton Hicks contractions	contractions felt in the womb during pregnancy from 16 weeks, which become more frequent towards full term.
Breech presentation	presentation of the buttocks of the fetus during labour.
Chorionic membrane	outer layer which forms the placenta.
Cyesis	pregnancy.
Embryo	the developing fertilised egg (first eight weeks of development while all rudimentary organs are forming).
Fetus	the developing baby after embryo stage until birth.
Fundus of uterus	the area of the uterus opposite its opening into the vagina (the top part).
Gestation	period of pregnancy.
Grand multipara	woman who has given birth to several children from different pregnancies.
Gravida	pregnant woman.
Gynaecologist	specialist in diseases of the female reproductive system.
Gynaecology	study of the female reproductive system.
Involution	return of the womb to its normal size following the baby's birth.
Lactation	production of milk.
Linea nigra	pigmented line on abdomen in pregnancy.
Multigravida	woman who has been pregnant more than once.
Multipara	woman who has had more than one child.
Neonatal period	the four-week period following the baby's birth (pertaining to the baby).
Neonate	first four weeks of a baby's life.
Nullipara	woman who has never given birth.

Obstetrics	medicine concerned with pregnancy and childbirth.	**Cervical erosion**	of the neck of the womb.
Para 1	see Primipara.	**Cervical polyp**	a stalk-like benign tumour in the cervix.
Parturition	giving birth.	**Cervicitis**	inflammation of the neck of the womb.
Placenta praevia	the placenta is the presenting part for birth - antepartum haemorrhage occurs - caesarean section is essential in comlete placenta praevia.	**Chlamydia**	an infection of the vagina.
		Chloasma	patchy brown pigmentation on face (like a mask) appearing in pregnancy due to hormone changes - also in women on contraceptive pill.
Primigravida	woman in her first pregnancy.		
Primipara	woman who has given birth to a first child.		
Pudenda	external genital area.	**Chorion epithelioma**	malignant tumour of chorionic (embryo) cells usually after formation of hyatidiform mole complication.
Puerperium	period of six weeks for mother following the birth of baby.		
Retroverted uterus	backward tilting of the womb.		
Trimester of pregnancy	a three-month period of pregnancy, e.g. first three months.	**Cryptomenorrhoea**	hidden menstruation - loss remains inside the womb due to an unbroken hymen.
Viable	capable of independent life (i.e. the fetus from 24 weeks of pregnancy).	**Cystic fibrosis**	inherited disease in which glandular tissue abnormal and, in particular, lung tissue becomes increasingly unable to function properly.

DISEASES AND DISORDERS

Amenorrhoea	absence of menstruation.		
Anaplasia	highly malignant cells.	**Cystocele**	prolapse of the base of the bladder in women; causes bulging of the wall of the vagina.
Antepartum haemorrhage	abnormal bleeding from the womb before the birth.		
Bartholin's abscess	painful collection of pus in the Bartholin's glands of the vulva.	**Dermoid cyst**	congenital (present at birth) sac containing embryonic tissue of hair, nails, teeth, skin etc.
Bicornuate uterus	abnormality where womb has two cavities.		
Caput succedaneum	soft swelling caused by free fluid (oedema) on the head of a newborn baby at, or shortly after, birth - disappears rapidly.	**Down's syndrome**	congenital condition in which there is often severe mental abnormality together with physical features of a mongoloid appearance, large tongue and stubby hands (abnormality of chromosome 21).
Carneous mole	pregnancy ceases and products of conception are retained in the womb.		

Dysfunctional uterine bleeding — heavy menstrual bleeding which does not appear to have any anatomical cause

Dysmenorrhoea — painful periods.

Dyspareunia — painful intercourse.

Dystocia — slow, difficult labour.

Eclampsia — a condition in which fits occur as blood pressure becomes extremely high (danger to both fetus and mother, see pre-eclampsia).

Ectopic pregnancy — embedding of fertilised egg outside of the womb - usually in the fallopian tube.

Endometriosis — condition where lining of womb is found in other sites, e.g. colon or pouch of Douglas.

Fibroadenoma — a benign tumour composed of fibrous and glandular tissue.

Fibroid — a benign tumour composed of fibrous and muscle tissue found in the womb.

Fibromyoma — a fibroid (as above).

Galactocele — milk cyst.

Gynaecomastia — enlargement of the male breast.

Hydatidiform mole — An intrauterine neoplastic mass.

Hydramnios — excessive amount of amniotic fluid.

Hyperemesis gravidarum — excessive vomiting during pregnancy.

Leucorrhoea — whitish vaginal discharge.

Leukoplakia vulva — chronic condition characterised by thick, hard, white patches on the vulva.

Lochia — vaginal discharge following childbirth.

Malpresentation — abnormal presentation of fetus for delivery.

Mastitis — inflammation of the breast.

Mastodynia — pain in the breast.

Meconium — first fetal stools - if passed in the womb it is a clear indication of fetal distress in labour.

Menorrhagia — excessive loss of blood during menstruation.

Metritis — inflammation of the womb.

Metrorrhagia — heavy bleeding not at the time of a period.

Metrostaxis — persistent slight bleeding from the womb.

Miscarriage — spontaneous abortion.

Munchausen syndrome by proxy — a situation where a child or other person is deliberately made to appear ill or suffer injury so that the person responsible gains attention.

Oligohydramnios — scanty amniotic fluid.

Polymenorrhoea — frequent periods.

Post-partum haemorrhage — bleeding following delivery.

Pre-eclampsia — a condition during pregnancy where there is a raised blood pressure, albumin in the urine and oedema of the face and body (also known as **toxaemia of pregnancy**) - it precedes eclampsia.

Procidentia — complete prolapse of womb into vagina through to the outside of the body.

Prolapse — womb or vaginal wall protrudes into the vagina.

Pseudocyesis — false pregnancy.

Puerperal psychosis — severe mental illness following childbirth.

Puerperal sepsis — infection of the genital tract and blood poisoning following childbirth.

Pyosalpingitis — inflammation of the fallopian tube with pus formation.

Pyosalpinx — presence of pus in the fallopian tube.

Rectocele — prolapse of the rectum into the vaginal wall.

Salpingitis	inflammation of the fallopian tubes.
Striae gravidarum	silvery lines (red at first) on thighs and abdomen occurring due to pregnancy - 'stretch marks'.
Supernumerary nipples	development of extra nipples (male or female).
Teratogenic	'monster producing'- a virus or factor which is capable of producing deformities in the developing fetus, e.g. drugs/rubella.
Vaginismus	involuntary spasm of the vagina preventing penetration during sexual intercourse.
Vaginitis	inflammation of the vagina.

PROCEDURES AND EQUIPMENT

Abortion	miscarriage or expulsion of the 'products of conception' from the uterus before 24 weeks:
Criminal a.	not within the legal definition;
Induced a.	intentional abortion;
Incomplete a.	parts of 'products of conception' are still remaining in the womb;
Inevitable a.	profuse bleeding, cervix dilated - products are bound to be expelled;
Spontaneous a.	naturally occurring abortion;
Threatened a.	slight bleeding (cervix closed).
Amniocentesis	withdrawal of the amniotic fluid which surrounds the developing fetus for examination purposes, e.g. for Down's syndrome.
Apgar score/rating	an estimation of the state of the newborn baby one minute after birth and again five minutes later - respiration, colour, muscle tone, pulse and response are measured with a maximum score of 10 being awarded for a healthy condition.
Caesarian section	delivery of fetus through abdominal incision.
Chorionic villus sampling	a sampling of cells from the chorion layer of the developing embryo for diagnostic purposes (can be done earlier than amniocentesis).
Colporrhaphy	surgical repair of vaginal wall prolapse.
Cone biopsy	cone-shaped portion of tissue removed from cervix for microscopic examination.
Endometrial smear/biopsy	following a small amount of local anaesthetic a thin, hollow curette is inserted through the cervical os and a small amount of uterine lining is removed for histology.
Epidural	injection of anaesthesia into meninges of lumbar spine, used to remove pain of childbirth.
Episiotomy	cutting the perineum (area between the vaginal opening and anus) to facilitate birth.
Fine needle aspiration	aspiration of breast lump, etc. for cytological investigation.
Guthrie test	blood test to detect **phenylketonuria** performed on newborn after establishment of feeding ('heel prick test').
Hysterectomy	surgical removal of the uterus which may be performed vaginally or by abdominal

incision.

Hysterotomy cutting into the womb.

Induction causing labour to begin by artificial means.

Lumpectomy (tilectomy) surgical removal of a tumour without removal of the breast itself.

Mammogram (phy) an X-ray procedure examining breast tissue.

Mastectomy surgical removal of the breast.

Myomectomy surgical removal of fibroids.

Oestradiol - 17β test for ovarian function.

Oophorectomy surgical removal of the ovary - (**bilateral oophorectomy** - both ovaries).

Panhysterectomy surgical removal of womb and surrounding reproductive organs.

Salpingectomy surgical removal of the fallopian tube(s).

Salpingo-oophorectomy surgical removal of ovary and fallopian tube.

Salpingogram X-ray of the fallopian tubes.

Thermography investigation of the breast by measuring the heat of the tissues.

Tilectomy see Lumpectomy.

Version turning of a fetus to aid delivery.

Vulvectomy surgical removal of the vulva.

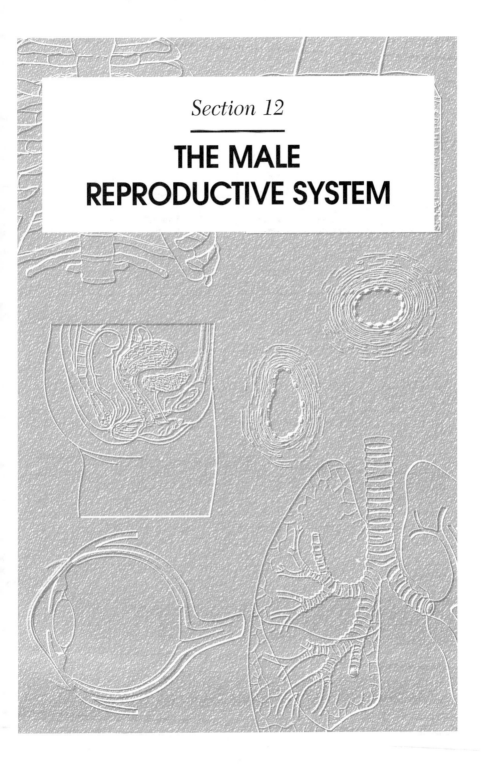

Section 12

THE MALE
REPRODUCTIVE SYSTEM

STRUCTURE

This system is composed of (see Figure 40):

- Two **testes**
- Two **epididymides** } within the scrotum
- Two **vasa deferentia**
- Two **seminal vesicles**
- **Prostate gland**
- Two **ejaculatory ducts**
- **Bulbourethral (Cowper's) glands**
- **Penis** containing the **urethra**

Testes

These develop within the abdominal cavity in the fetus, but prior to birth they descend through a canal known as the **inguinal canal** into the **scrotum**. They produce numerous **spermatazoa** (male sex cells) for fertilisation of the female ovum. Also produced are the male hormones known as **androgens**, the main one being **testosterone**, which are responsible for secondary male characteristics (hair distribution etc).

Scrotum

The scrotum is a pouch of skin and specialised tissue lying outside the abdominal cavity and containing the **testis** and **epididymis**, together with the attached start of the **vas deferens**. It is essential that the developing **spermatazoa** are kept at a temperature lower than that within the abdominal cavity where the organs were first developed in fetal life. Unless this occurs the man will be **infertile**. The scrotum is lowered from and raised closer to the body, by special muscles dependent on the temperature of blood passing through the structure.

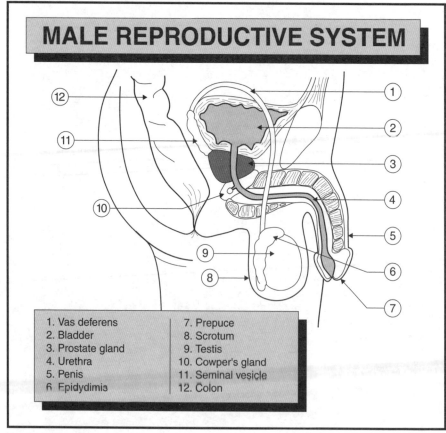

MALE REPRODUCTIVE SYSTEM

1. Vas deferens	7. Prepuce
2. Bladder	8. Scrotum
3. Prostate gland	9. Testis
4. Urethra	10. Cowper's gland
5. Penis	11. Seminal vesicle
6. Epidydimis	12. Colon

Figure 40 - The male reproductive system.

Epididymides

These are situated upon the testes; here the immobile **spermatazoa** become mature and are stored.

Vasa deferentia

Tubes through which the spermatazoa are released. These are cut in the operation of **vasectomy** to produce sterilisation of the male.

Seminal vesicles

These contribute their own secretion to the seminal fluid which keeps the spermatazoa active and alive. Some spermatazoa are stored here ready for **ejaculation**.

Ejaculatory ducts

These join the seminal vesicles to the urethra.

Bulbourethral glands

These are also known as **Cowper's glands** and produce further secretions to the seminal fluid.

Prostate gland

A gland the size of a walnut surrounding the junction of the vasa deferentia and urethra. It secretes a fluid making the spermatazoa more mobile and fertile. It commonly becomes enlarged in older men causing difficulty in passing urine due to constriction of the urethra.

Urethra

This is a common passageway for both **seminal fluid** and **urine**. A **sphincter muscle** prevents both functions occurring at the same time.

Penis

This is the male organ composed of **erectile** tissue and capable of becoming erect when distended with blood. The enlargement at its tip is known as the **glans**; the fold of skin protecting the opening of the urethra is known as the **foreskin** or **prepuce** and it is this area which is removed in the procedure of **circumcision**.

ABBREVIATIONS

HPV	human papilloma virus
PSA	prostatic specific antigen (test for cancer of prostate)
TUR	transurethral resection (of prostate gland)
TURB	transurethral resection of bladder
TURBT	transurethral resection of bladder tumour
TURP	transurethral resection of prostate gland

TERMINOLOGY

Andr/o	stem for male.
Epididym/o	stem for epididymis (fine tubules).
Genit/o	stem for genital.
Orchi(d)/o	stem for testis.
Phall/o (pen/o)	stem for penis.
Prostat/o	stem for prostate gland.
Semin/o	stem for semen.
Vas/o	stem for vas deferens.

DISEASES AND DISORDERS

Balanitis	inflammation of glans penis and foreskin.
Ectopic testes	testicles which are in the wrong place, i.e. not in the scrotum.
Epididymitis	inflammation of the epididymis (tubules above the testis).
Epididymo-orchitis	inflammation of the epididymis and testis.
Epispadias	opening of urethra on the upper side of penis.
Haematocele	effusion of blood in area surrounding the testis.
Hydrocele	collection of fluid in the tunica vaginalis (membrane surrounding the testis).
Hypospadias	opening of urethra is on the lower side of the penis.
Impotence	inability to have sexual intercourse, or the inability to have or maintain an erection of the penis (may have a physical or a psychological cause).
Orchitis (orchiditis)	inflammation of a testicle.

Phallitis	inflammation of the penis.	**Orchidopexy**	fixing of an undescended or rotating testicle into the scrotal sac.
Phimosis	constriction of foreskin of penis preventing retraction of skin.	**Prostatic specific antigen test**	this is a screening blood test used to aid diagnosis of carcinoma of the prostate gland. Patients with prostatism (enlargement of the prostate gland) should be screened in order to eliminate the possibility of malignancy.
Prostatitis	inflammation of the prostate gland.		
Sterility	inability to fertilise female egg (ovum).		
Urethritis	inflammation of the urethra.		
Varicocele	dilatation of veins around the testis and vas deferens.		

PROCEDURES AND EQUIPMENT

Circumcision	surgical removal of part of foreskin.	**Suprapubic cystostomy**	incision above the prostate to allow drainage of the bladder.
Ileal conduit	ureters are transplanted into the ileum (intestine) in order to discharge urine to bypass a tumour or following removal of bladder.	**Transurethral resection of prostate**	(TURP) surgical removal of the prostate through the urethra.
		Urethroplasty	reshaping of the urethra.
Orchidectomy	surgical removal of a testicle.	**Vasectomy**	surgical cutting/ removal of the vasa deferentia in order to produce sterility.

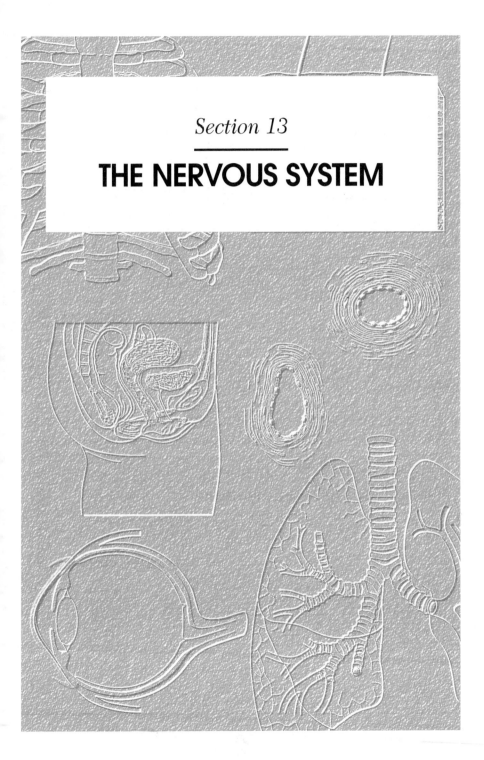

Section 13

THE NERVOUS SYSTEM

FUNCTION

This is concerned with the rapid conduction and interpretation of messages in the form of electrical impulses from one part of the body to another. It also co-ordinates the activities of the body.

STRUCTURE

The nervous system is made up of specialised tissue containing cells known as neurones, and is divided into three systems:

- **Central nervous system** (CNS)
- **Peripheral nervous system**
- **Autonomic nervous system** (ANS)

Nerve cells are known as **grey matter** and the fibres from them are covered in **myelin** (a fatty substance) **white matter**. In the CNS, nerve cells, when damaged, are unable to regenerate themselves.

Messages can only travel in one direction along a nerve fibre.

Motor nerves (efferent)

These convey messages from the brain to parts of the body to perform an action (see Figure 41).

Sensory nerves (afferent)

These convey messages from the body to the brain with information about stimuli such as pain.

CENTRAL NERVOUS SYSTEM

This consists of the **brain** and **spinal cord**.

BRAIN

The brain lies within the bony **cranium** of the skull. It is covered in a specialised membrane containing the blood vessels which supply oxygen and nourishment, known as the **meninges**, which also covers the spinal cord. The need for oxygen to every cell in the brain is critical. If deprived of oxygen for more than three to four minutes, these cells will die and death will occur.

The brain consists of (see Figure 42):

- **Cerebrum**
- **Cerebellum**
- **Brain stem**

Cerebrum

This forms the larger lobes of the brain and is divided into two **hemispheres** joined together with a bridge of white matter. The cerebrum contains the **higher centres** including those of intellect, consciousness, movement, sensory perception etc.

There are many specialised centres and the **convoluted** surface, together with numerous **fissures** (giving a larger surface area), contains **grey matter**, with **white matter** within

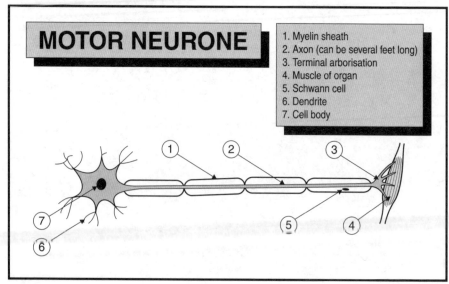

MOTOR NEURONE

1. Myelin sheath
2. Axon (can be several feet long)
3. Terminal arborisation
4. Muscle of organ
5. Schwann cell
6. Dendrite
7. Cell body

Figure 41 - A motor neurone.

the hemispheres. There are also specialised areas of grey matter deep within the hemispheres known as the **basal ganglia**. The **hypothalamus**, which controls the ANS, is situated here.

The **cerebrum** consists of numerous **lobes** which are named from the cranial bones beneath which they lie, i.e. **frontal**, **parietal**, **temporal** and **occipital**.

Cerebellum

This also has two hemispheres joined together at the posterior portion. It is involved in the control of **muscle tone** and co-ordinates muscular movement as well as balance and equilibrium. Damage can cause **ataxia** (unco-ordinated gait), tremor and loss of sense of balance.

Brainstem

This consists of:

- **Midbrain**
- **Pons varolii**
- **Medulla oblongata**

} all interconnected

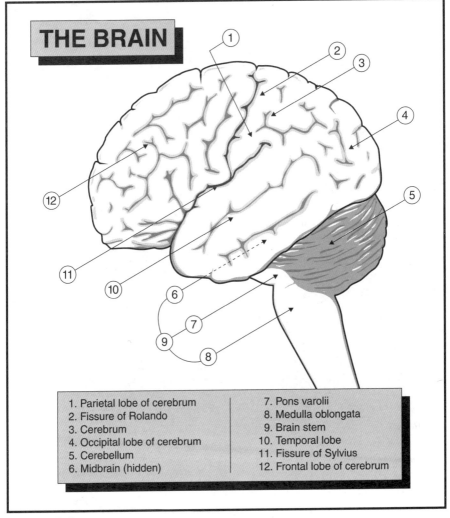

THE BRAIN

1. Parietal lobe of cerebrum
2. Fissure of Rolando
3. Cerebrum
4. Occipital lobe of cerebrum
5. Cerebellum
6. Midbrain (hidden)
7. Pons varolii
8. Medulla oblongata
9. Brain stem
10. Temporal lobe
11. Fissure of Sylvius
12. Frontal lobe of cerebrum

Figure 42 - The brain.

Midbrain

This joins the two cerebral hemispheres to the **cerebellum** and the **pons varolii** below. It has specialised centres deep within it. All sensory impulses pass through this area.

Pons varolii

This joins the **cerebellum** to the **midbrain** and **medulla oblongata** below.

Medulla oblongata

This is continuous with the pons above and contains the **vital centres**, including the control of respiration, heart beat and the calibre of the blood vessels etc.

Damage to these centres is very serious and often causes death, e.g. fracture of the base of the skull. This area is continuous with the spinal cord below and passes through the **foramen magnum** (large hole) of the cranium.

It is in the medulla oblongata that the white nerve fibres, travelling to the spinal cord, cross over so that the left area of the brain controls the right side of the body and *vice versa*.

Ventricles

Deep within the brain are spaces known as **ventricles**, which are continuous with each other and with the fine spinal canal in the spinal cord. **Cerebrospinal fluid** from the **meninges** circulates throughout these areas.

Meninges

This is a very specialised membrane which covers both brain and spinal cord.

It is composed of three special layers:

1. **Dura mater**   a hard, tough outer layer.
2. **Arachnoid mater**   a vascular layer with many blood vessels.
3. **Pia mater**   a soft layer closely attached to brain and spinal cord

Functions

It has the following functions:

- **Supports** the delicate nervous tissue.
- Acts as a **shock absorber**.
- Maintains **uniform pressure** around it.
- Provides **nourishment** and removes **waste products**.

Cranial nerves

The 12 pairs of cranial nerves arising from the brain, are sensory and motor. **Motor nerves** carry messages *from* the brain *to* the body and **sensory nerves** carry messages *to* the brain *from* the body.

List of cranial nerves

m = motor   s = sensory

I **olfactory**	concerning sense of smell. (s)
II **optic**	concerning sight. (s)
III **oculomotor**	eye muscles. (m)
IV **trochlear**	eye muscles. (m)
V **trigeminal**	forehead and face. (s)
VI **abducens**	eye muscles. (m)
VII **facial**	facial expression. (m)
VIII **auditory**	hearing and balance. (s)
IX **glossopharyngeal**	tongue and pharynx. (ms)
X **vagus** (**vagal**)	pharynx, trachea, heart, larynx, bronchi lungs, oesophagus, stomach, intestine. (ms)
XI **spinal accessory**	muscles of pharynx etc. (m)
XII **hypoglossal**	muscles of tongue. (m)

SPINAL CORD
Structure

This is continuous with the **medulla oblongata** above and extends to the level of the **second lumbar vertebra** below. It travels through the **neural canal** or **foramen** (hole) in the vertebrae which surround and protect it.

Unlike the brain, the grey matter of the spinal cord is found deep within it in an H-shaped pattern and the white matter distributed in the outer aspects. It is covered in **meninges** and has a small space through its centre, known as the **spinal canal**.

Arising from the spinal cord are the **peripheral nerves** of which there are 31 pairs, travelling to the various parts of the body, receiving and sending messages and interconnecting.

A group of nerve fibres (**white matter**) travelling together is known as a **plexus** and groups of cells (**grey matter**) as **ganglia**.

At the termination of the spinal cord (at the level of the second lumbar vertebra in the adult) numerous peripheral nerves give rise to the **cauda equina** (**horse's tail**) which supply the **lumbar-sacral** area (in the groin) and lower limbs (see Figure 43).

Function

Its function is to relay messages to and from the body and also at different levels of the cord itself.

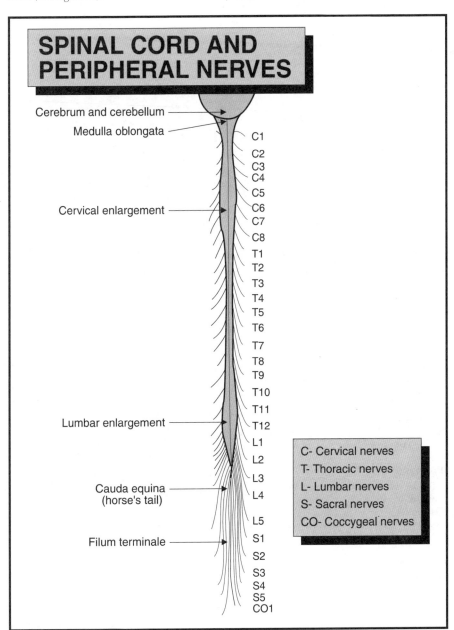

SPINAL CORD AND PERIPHERAL NERVES

Cerebrum and cerebellum

Medulla oblongata

C1
C2
C3
C4
C5

Cervical enlargement — C6
C7
C8
T1
T2
T3
T4
T5
T6
T7
T8
T9
T10
T11

Lumbar enlargement — T12
L1
L2

Cauda equina (horse's tail) — L3
L4
L5

Filum terminale — S1
S2
S3
S4
S5
CO1

C- Cervical nerves
T- Thoracic nerves
L- Lumbar nerves
S- Sacral nerves
CO- Coccygeal nerves

Figure 43 - The spinal cord and peripheral nerves.

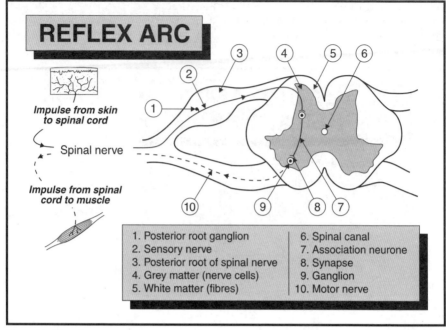

REFLEX ARC

Impulse from skin to spinal cord

Spinal nerve

Impulse from spinal cord to muscle

1. Posterior root ganglion
2. Sensory nerve
3. Posterior root of spinal nerve
4. Grey matter (nerve cells)
5. White matter (fibres)
6. Spinal canal
7. Association neurone
8. Synapse
9. Ganglion
10. Motor nerve

Figure 44 - The reflex arc.

Reflex action

This is the automatic reaction by the body to a stimulation. In a **reflex arc**, a message to the sensory area of the spinal cord is immediately relayed across the cord to the **motor area**, which in turn sends an impulse to a **motor organ**, e.g. a muscle. The original sensory message still travels to the appropriate part of the brain, but the resulting movement of the limb is started more quickly by the reflex action, i.e. the reaction of the body to a pinprick of the arm is a reflex arc that moves the arm (see Figure 44).

Inhibition

This is where the resulting reflex action is overcome by the brain, e.g. picking up a very hot plate which is very expensive. The automatic dropping of the plate is overridden by the knowledge that it is expensive to replace.

PERIPHERAL NERVOUS SYSTEM

This consists of:

- 12 pairs of **cranial nerves**
- 31 pairs of **peripheral nerves**

The cranial nerves arise from the brain itself. The peripheral nerves stem from differing levels of the spinal cord and supply the body. They convey sensory and motor impulses to and from the brain and spinal cord, and also to different levels of the cord itself.

AUTONOMIC NERVE SUPPLY

This is the system which controls the workings of the body organs and keeps the body in its correct state (**homeostasis**). It is not normally within the control of the will but is automatic.

It supplies all organs composed of **smooth muscle** as well as other organs, including the heart, blood vessels, respiratory system and eyes. There are two sets of fibres to each organ which are known as the:

- **sympathetic** chain
- **parasympathetic** chain

These are controlled by a centre in the brain known as the **hypothalamus**. All systems work in conjunction with each other and the two sets of fibres work in harmony.

Sympathetic chain

This set of fibres is stimulated to prepare the body for the '**fight or flight**' response. When stimulated, it increases the heart rate and respiration, raises blood pressure, dilates the pupil of the eye and increases energy supplies as well as many other actions.

Parasympathetic chain

This set of fibres has an inhibiting or resting action and has the opposite effect upon the body to the sympathetic chain. Its action slows the heart rate, decreases the breathing rate and increases digestion and secretion of saliva.

The **vagus nerve**, as part of the parasympathetic chain, supplies the heart and many of the major organs of the body.

ABBREVIATIONS

ADD	attention deficit disorder
ANS	autonomic nervous system
BSE	bovine spongiform encephalopathy ('mad cow' disease)
CA	chronological age
CAT (CT) scan	computerised X-ray of layers of tissues
CJD	Creutzfeldt–Jacob disease
CNS	central nervous system
CSF	cerebrospinal fluid
CVA	cerebrovascular accident (stroke)
DS	disseminated sclerosis (old term for MS)
DTs	delirium tremens
ECT	electroconvulsive therapy
EEG	electroencephalogram
EMG	electromyogram
GA	general anaesthetic
GPI	general paralysis of the insane
IQ	intelligence quotient
LA	local anaesthetic
MA	mental age
MAOI	monoamine oxidase inhibitors (antidepressants which require abstinence from certain foods, e.g. cheese - can cause bleeding in the brain)
MND	motor neurone disease
MRI	magnetic resonance imaging (see NMR)
MS	multiple sclerosis
NMR	nuclear magnetic resonance (scan)
nvCJD	new variant Creutzfeldt–Jacob disease
OCD	obsessive compulsive disorder
REM	rapid eye movements
RT	radiation therapy
RTA	road traffic accident
SADS	seasonal affective disorder syndrome (depression due to lack of light in winter)
SAH	subarachnoid haemorrhage
SOL	space-occupying lesion (tumour, usually malignant, in the cranium)
SSRI	selective serotonin reuptake inhibitor (antidepressants which affect particular enzyme actions in brain)
TCA	tricyclic antidepressant (old type of antidepressant)
TENS	transcutaneous electrical nerve stimulation
TIA	transient ischaemic attack (in the brain)
TLE	temporal lobe epilepsy (fits which originate in the temporal lobe of brain causing aura of taste, hearing, smell etc.)

COMMON SUFFIXES

-paresis	weakness
-phasia	speech
-plegia	paralysis

TERMINOLOGY

Cephal/o	stem for head.
Cerebell/o	stem for cerebellum (part of the brain).
Cerebr/o	stem for cerebrum (part of the brain).
Crani/o	cranium.
Encephal/o	brain.
Myel/o	spinal cord.
Neur/o	stem for nerve.

Poli/o	grey matter.
Psych/o	mind/behaviour.
Ventricul/o	ventricles of brain.
Catharsis	an outlet of repressed emotion.
Cognitive behaviour psychology	person's treatment which concentrates on changing behaviour instead of the actual cause of the problem.
Complex	a pattern of behaviour which demonstrates an over-reaction to a problem.
Cerebrospinal fluid	fluid similar to plasma found in the meninges which nourishes the brain and spinal cord.
Delusion	false belief, usually associated with psychological illness, which cannot be altered despite logic and evidence to the contrary.
Dura mater	outermost and thickest of the three meninges surrounding brain and spinal chord.
Perception	the interpretation and response of the nervous system to sensory stimuli.
Psychiatrist	medical specialist in mental illness.
Psychiatry	the medical speciality concerning mental illness.
Psychoanalysis	Freudian method of exploring the mind.
Psychologist	specialist in the study of behaviour, including the normal - not medically qualified.
Psychology	scientific study of behaviour.
Psychotherapy	treatment by psychological methods.

DISEASES AND DISORDERS

Affective disorders	those conditions which affect mood.
Affective psychosis	major mental disorder in which there is serious disturbance of the emotions.
Alzheimer's disease	progressive dementia - caused by destruction of the neurones (brain cells).
Amnesia	loss of memory.
Anaesthesia	loss of sensitivity and feeling (local) to a part or (general) throughout the body, causing loss of consciousness.
Anencephaly	partial or complete absence of the bones of the rear of the skull and of the cerebral hemispheres of the brain.
Anorexia nervosa	eating disorder characterised by refusal to eat - person has body image of obesity (common in teenage girls).
Aphasia	inability to speak caused by brain damage.
Apoplexy	a stroke.
Ataxia	unco-ordinated gait (limp).
Aura	warning symptoms preceding epileptic seizure or migraine attack.
Autism	absorption with the self - a condition in which the person is withdrawn into their own world, showing little response to events around them.
Babinski's sign	reflex of the toe upwards instead of down - shows damage to central nervous system (CNS).
Bell's palsy	paralysis of face muscles due to injury or disease of cranial nerve supplying face muscles (usually one-sided).
Bovine spongiform encephalopathy	see Creutzfeldt–Jacob disease.

Bulimia nervosa	eating disorder characterised by eating 'binges' and vomiting.	**Delirium tremens**	mental excitement due to chronic excessive alcohol intake, known as 'DTs'.
Catatonia	state of stupor, strange posture, outbursts of excitement - form of autism common in schizophrenia.	**Depression**	an intense long-term lowering of mood and function.
Causalgia	severe burning-type pain caused by nerve injury.	*Endogenous*	caused by internal body factors, as in manic depression where there are alternating mood swings to intense euphoria.
Chorea	involuntary contraction of muscles causing writhing movements (St Vitus' dance).	*Exogenous or reactive*	caused by events and environmental factors, e.g. bereavement or unemployment.
Clonus response	the production of a series of muscle contractions in response to a stimulus which are only produced in the presence of CNS (central nervous system) disease.	*Involutional*	caused by ageing process including menopause.
		Diplopia	double vision.
		Dysarthria	difficulty in articulation of speech due to nerve damage.
Coma	complete unconsciousness - a level where there is no response on normal stimulation.	**Dyskinesia**	abnormal movements associated with side-effects of major tranquillising drugs.
Compression	pressure on the brain tissue due to swelling, blood clot or tumour.	**Dyslexia**	word blindness - inability to decipher words by the brain producing difficulty in reading, writing etc, by an individual with the intelligence to perform these tasks.
Concussion	limited period of unconsciousness caused by injury to the head.		
Coning	pressure on brain forcing brainstem through foramen magnum.		
Creutzfeldt–Jacob disease	a disease in which the brain tissue degenerates; linked with bovine spongiform encephalopathy (mad cow disease) it is now known to be transmitted to humans.	**Dysthymia**	depression associated with imaginary illness.
		Encephalitis	inflammation of the brain.
		Epilepsy	condition of suffering seizures, convulsions - abnormal electrical activity of the brain.
		Idiopathic epilepsy	epilepsy of unknown cause.
		Jacksonian epilepsy	epilepsy having a focal area - caused by an abnormality in that area of the brain, e.g. scar tissue.
Delirium	mental excitement resulting from hallucinations, e.g. in state of high fever, alcohol consumption, or mental illness.	*Post-epileptic automatism*	a period following a fit when the person functions automatically and is unaware of their actions.

Petit mal	type of epilepsy where the person momentarily loses concentration ('absences').
Grand mal	attacks which include loss of consciousness and convulsions where the disturbance in electrical activity spreads across the various areas of the brain.
Convulsion	spasmodic contraction and relaxation of muscles in a fit.
Status epilepticus	a continuous fit passing from one straight into another - very dangerous.
Fixation	an arrest in psychological development at a particular stage.
Fugue	period of altered awareness often associated with wandering, of which the person has no recall.
General paralysis of the insane	paralysis caused by the terminal effects of syphilis.
Glioma	malignant tumour of nerve support system.
Grand mal	see Epilepsy.
Hallucination	false perception without any true sensory stimuli - any sense may be involved, e.g. taste, hearing, sight etc.
Hemianaesthesia	loss of feeling of one side of the body.
Hemiparaesthesia	heightened sensation of one side of the body.
Hemiparesis	weakness of one side of the body.
Hemiplegia	paralysis of one side of the body.
Herpes zoster	shingles - painful infection along the nerve by the virus which causes chickenpox.
Hydrocephaly	'water on the brain' - excess cerebrospinal fluid present due to a blockage in its circulation - skull enlarges in the baby.

Hyperkinetic	overactivity of movement.
Hypochondria	an abnormality in which the person is pre-occupied with imaginary illnesses.
Hysteria	a neurosis arising from psychological problems producing bodily symptoms, e.g. paralysis.
Kernig's sign	inability to straighten leg at knee joint when thigh is flexed at right angles to the body - present in meningitis.
Libido	sexual energy/ behaviour/drive.
Mania	abnormal elevation of the mood and overactivity.
Manic depression	a form of depression which is characterised by alternating mood swings of overactivity (mania) and sadness (depression) - a psychosis; see Depression, endogenous.
Meningioma	tumour of the meninges (covering of the brain and spinal cord).
Meningism	irritation of the meninges (covering of the brain and spinal cord).
Meningitis	inflammation of the meninges.
Meningocele	protrusion of the meninges through the gap in the unfused vertebra of spina bifida.
Microcephaly	having an abnormally small head.
Migraine	headache, often one-sided, characterised by disturbance of vision nausea, vomiting etc, caused by dilatation of the cranial arteries.
Monoplegia	paralysis of one limb.
Motor neurone disease	disease of the motor areas of the central

nervous system causing paralysis - rapidly progressive.

Multiple sclerosis   disease of central nervous system in which the myelin (fatty) sheath covering nerve fibres is destroyed and various functions are impaired, including movement. It is characterised by relapses and remissions.

Myelitis   inflammation of the spinal cord.

Myelomeningocele   meningocele where the spinal cord is also protruding.

Narcolepsy   compulsive sleeping (at any time).

Neuralgia   nerve pain (along the course of a nerve).

Neuritis   inflammation of a nerve.

Neurosis   a form of mental illness of which the (neurotic) patient has insight (awareness that they are ill), anxiety and depression.

Nystagmus   involuntary rapid movements of the eyeballs.

Palsy   paralysis.

Panic attacks   present in anxiety states - body response produces rapid heart rate etc.

Paranoia   a state in which person suffers unfounded (paranoid) feelings of persecution.

Paraplegia   paralysis of both legs.

Paresis   weakness.

Parkinson's disease   damage to grey matter in the brain known as the basal ganglia; causes involuntary tremors of limbs etc.

Petit mal   see Epilepsy.

Phobia   irrational fear.

Photophobia   intolerance of light.

Poliomyelitis   inflammation of the grey matter of the spinal cord (infantile paralysis).

Polyneuritis   inflammation of many nerves.

Psychopath   a person having no social conscience.

Psychosis   mental illness in which the patient has no insight (i.e. psychotic) - unaware that they are ill; affects the whole personality.

Romberg's sign   an inability to stand without swaying when the eyes are closed and the feet are together - sign of brain damage.

Schizoid   split personality - being more than one personality (**not** 'as in schizophrenia').

Schizophrenia   a psychosis of unknown cause in which the person suffers delusions and hallucinations - thought processes are disordered.

Sciatica   pain along the sciatic nerve (down the back of the leg to the toe).

Sinus thrombosis   formation of blood clot in the brain sinuses (spaces in which the venous blood drains before entering the jugular veins).

Spastic   damage to motor area of brain producing increased muscle tone.

St Vitus' dance   see Chorea.

Stupor   a level of consciousness - person not fully conscious but does respond to certain stimuli.

Subarachnoid haemorrhage   bleeding between the layers of the meninges known as the pia mater and the arachnoid mater.

Subdural haematoma   a blood clot between the layers of the meninges - the dura mater and the

mater and the
arachnoid mater.

Syncope fainting - temporary lack of blood to the brain.

Syphilis sexually transmitted disease which, in its final stages, produces damage to the central nervous system.

Tabes dorsalis (locomotor ataxia) nerve damage to the spinal cord caused by the late stages of syphilis and giving rise to an abnormal gait.

Tetraplegia (quadriplegia) paralysis of all four limbs.

Tremor involuntary quivering of the muscles - inability to control them.

Trigeminal neuralgia inflammation of the Vth cranial nerve supplying three areas of the face; causes severe pain.

Vertigo dizziness.

PROCEDURES AND EQUIPMENT

Cerebral angiogram X-ray demonstration of the blood vessels of the brain using an opaque dye.

Cisternal puncture same as lumbar puncture, but the needle is inserted into area at base of skull - used in investigation of cerebrospinal fluid (CSF) in children.

Craniotomy cutting into the bony cranium of the skull; used to relieve pressure etc.

Electroencephalogram a tracing which records the electrical activity of the brain (used in diagnosis of epilepsy, tumours and other brain conditions).

Electromyogram a tracing which records the electrical activity of muscles to show if there is any abnormality in the pattern of activity, both at rest and on movement.

Intrathecal injection directly into the meninges.

Lumbar puncture insertion of a needle into the meninges of the spinal cord to withdraw CSF for investigation.

Myelogram special X-ray using radio-opaque dye of the spinal cord.

Transcutaneous nerve stimulation a method of relieving chronic pain by electrical stimulation of other nerve endings.

Trephine instrument used for removing circular sections of tissue from skull area (trephining).

Ventriculogram X-ray demonstration of the ventricles of the brain. This procedure is being replaced by CT and MRI scans.

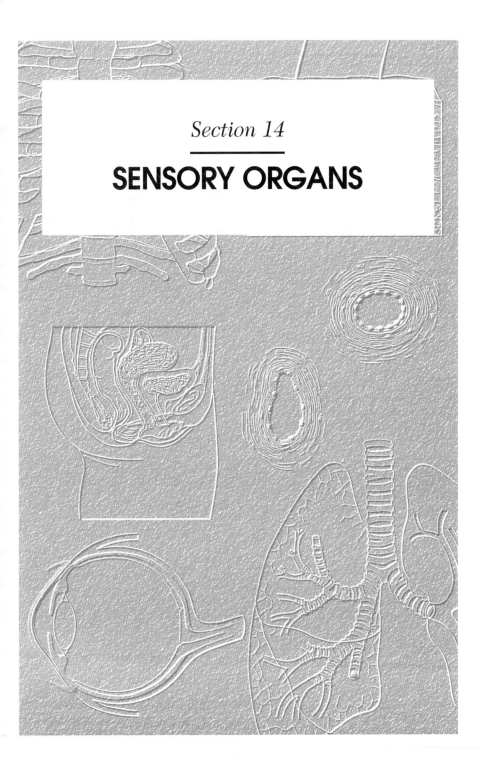

Section 14

SENSORY ORGANS

STRUCTURE

The special senses of the body consist of sight, hearing, smell, taste, touch, temperature and pain. The receptors for these senses are found in the following sensory organs:

- **eye**   sight
- **ear**   hearing and balance
- **nose**   smell
- **tongue**   taste
- **skin**   touch, temperature and pain (dealt with in Section 10)

THE EYE

The eye is the sensory organ of sight and is situated in the bony orbit of the skull which protects it. It receives messages which are conveyed to the brain for interpretation.

It consists of the following structures:

- **eyeball**
- appendages:
  - **eyebrows**
  - **eyelids**
  - **lacrimal apparatus** (tears)

EYEBALL

The eyeball is almost spherical in shape and is embedded in fat. It is protected at the front by eyebrows, eyelids and lashes, and is composed of three layers:

- **sclera**
- **choroid**
- **retina**

It also contains the **lens** and fluids known as the **aqueous** and **vitreous humour** which **refract** (bend) the rays of light to focus upon the retinal layer and form an image very similar to that within a camera (see Figure 45).

Sclera

This is the tough outer fibrous coat which helps to maintain the shape of the eyeball. Muscles are attached to it and the orbit, keeping it in place and enabling movement of the eyeball. The front part is covered in **conjunctiva**, a membrane which also lines the eyelids. At the front lies the cornea with which it is continuous.

Choroid

This is the vascular layer attached to the sclera, forming the middle layer of the eyeball. At the front of the eyeball it is continuous with the **ciliary body**, a muscular organ from which the lens is suspended, and the **iris**.

The iris is a pigmented muscular body with a hole in its centre which forms the **pupil**, through which light rays enter to focus upon the **retina** (nervous layer).

It is capable of constricting and relaxing, so altering the size of the pupil which controls the amount of light entering the eye.

Retina

This forms the inner layer of the eyeball and is attached to the choroid. It contains nerve fibres which are the origins of the **optic nerve** and include specialised light-sensitive structures known as **rods** and **cones**, which receive light and colour information for interpretation by the brain.

Rods receive sensations of light and dark, and are more numerous towards the front of the eye. Cones are concerned with sensations of colour. They are more numerous towards the back of the eyeball; red, green and blue are the prime colours for interpretation. **Colour blindness** arises from a lack or abnormality of these receptor cells.

The optic nerve, sheathed at the back of each eye, conveys the sensations from the retina to the **occipital** area of the brain for interpretation into sight. The nerve from each eye joins at an area known as the **optic chiasma**.

Macula (fovea)

This is an area of the retina where cones are most numerous and central vision most acute. It is immediately opposite the cornea.

Optic disc

This is the area where there are no rods or cones present, and is at the back of the eye where the optic nerve leaves the eyeball. It gives rise to an area known as the '**blind spot**', which is present in each field of vision. No sight is perceived from this area.

Optic fundus

This is an area including the **optic disc**, which can be examined by use of an **ophthalmoscope**. Changes to the retina and evidence of effects of high blood pressure or raised intra-cranial pressure, can be viewed in this way, enabling early diagnosis in some cases.

Muscles of the eyeball

There are three pairs attached to the sclera and the bony orbit, which enable movement of the

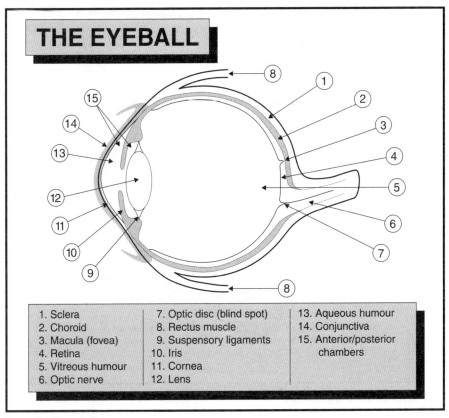

THE EYEBALL

1. Sclera	7. Optic disc (blind spot)	13. Aqueous humour
2. Choroid	8. Rectus muscle	14. Conjunctiva
3. Macula (fovea)	9. Suspensory ligaments	15. Anterior/posterior
4. Retina	10. Iris	chambers
5. Vitreous humour	11. Cornea	
6. Optic nerve	12. Lens	

Figure 45 - The eyeball.

eyeball. Normally the eyes move in unison which enables **binocular vision**. When the eyes move independently the condition produced is known as **strabismus** (squint). It is most important that any defect is diagnosed early in childhood as deficiency of sight can occur if treatment is delayed. Surgery and/or **orthoptic** exercises are used for correction.

Refraction

This is the term used for the bending of the light rays. It is necessary to ensure that images are focused upon the retina for clear vision. Images are perceived as **inverted** and are correctly interpreted by the brain. It is because of this that, in conditions of cerebral disturbance such as strokes and head injuries, vision is often disturbed. People who are **myopic** (short-sighted) tend to have a misshapen eyeball that is too long front to back, thus the images are in focus

in front of the retina. The opposite of this is **hypermetropia** (long-sightedness) where a visual defect means the light rays come to focus behind the retina as a result of the eyeball being too long top to bottom (see Figure 46). The structures involved in refraction are the:

- **cornea**
- **lens**
- **aqueous humour**
- **vitreous humour**

The cornea and lens, by their curvature, will bend light rays striking upon their surface.

Aqueous humour

This is a water-like fluid situated within the **anterior** and **posterior** chambers at the front of the eyeball.

Rays of light will also be bent while travelling through this substance.

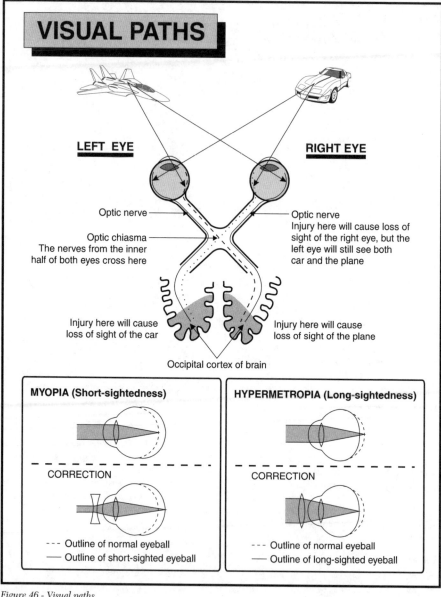

VISUAL PATHS

LEFT EYE

RIGHT EYE

Optic nerve

Optic chiasma
The nerves from the inner
half of both eyes cross here

Optic nerve
Injury here will cause loss of
sight of the right eye, but the
left eye will still see both
car and the plane

Injury here will cause
loss of sight of the car

Injury here will cause
loss of sight of the plane

Occipital cortex of brain

MYOPIA (Short-sightedness)

CORRECTION

--- Outline of normal eyeball
— Outline of short-sighted eyeball

HYPERMETROPIA (Long-sightedness)

CORRECTION

--- Outline of normal eyeball
— Outline of long-sighted eyeball

Figure 46 - Visual paths.

Vitreous humour

This is a thick jelly-like substance which fills the posterior portion of the eyeball (situated behind the lens) ensuring it maintains its shape. Light travelling through this substance is further bent to achieve focusing of images.

Pressure in the eyeball

In conditions of **glaucoma** where the aqueous humour fails to drain effectively, **intraocular pressure** is raised and damage to the retina occurs. In acute cases, urgent treatment is required to reduce this pressure if blindness is to be prevented.

Accommodation

This is the ability of the eye to focus near objects upon the retina. This is achieved by the alteration in the shape of the lens and its capsule by the constriction and relaxation of the **ciliary body** from which the lens is suspended. Ability to accommodate decreases with age as the elasticity of the lens and its capsule decreases.

Lacrimal apparatus

This consists of structures which produce tears:

- **Lacrimal gland**
- **Lacrimal ducts**
- **Lacrimal sac**
- **Nasolacrimal duct**

Tears consist of a slightly alkaline, salty fluid. These have a slightly antiseptic action and also keep the eyeball moist. They are involved in the expression of emotion.

THE EAR

This is the receptor organ of hearing and balance. Sound waves travel through the organ conveying messages to the brain for interpretation.

There are three main parts to the ear:

- External ear
- Middle ear
- Inner ear

External ear

This consists of the **auricle** or **pinna**, attached to the side of the head, and the **auditory canal**. The pinna acts like an ear trumpet to receive sound waves and is composed of skin and elastic cartilage.

The auditory canal within the skull carries sound waves from the pinna to the eardrum (**tympanic membrane**) which separates it from the middle ear. It is lined with skin containing hair and modified glands, which produce wax (**cerumen**) to protect the delicate membrane. If excessive wax is produced, deafness can occur because of the obstruction to the eardrum, preventing vibration. This wax may be removed by **syringing**.

Middle ear

This consists of a cavity within the temporal bone of the skull, filled with air and lined with mucous membrane. A canal known as the **eustachian tube** extends from the middle ear into the back of the nose (**naso-pharynx**) and it is through this, when swallowing occurs, that air is conducted, so ensuring an equal pressure between the external and middle ear.

Infection present in the nose or throat can easily spread to the middle ear, causing inflammation (**otitis media**), which in turn can cause **mastoiditis** (inflammation of the bone cells of the temporal bone of the skull). This can also lead to a brain abscess. It is for this reason that any infection must be treated as quickly as possible.

Ossicles

These are three tiny bony structures named from their shapes of hammer (**malleus**), anvil (**incus**) and stirrup (**stapes**). They are attached in a chain by ligaments, allowing them to vibrate causing the conduction of sound waves from the **tympanic membrane** into the **inner ear**.

The malleus is connected to the tympanic membrane and the stapes to the oval window (**fenestra ovalis**) of the inner ear. Each of these two ossicles is attached to the incus (see Figure 47).

Inner ear

This is situated within the bony labyrinth of the temporal bone. It consists of numerous bony canals and cavities. It is lined with a membrane known as the **membranous labyrinth** and is filled with fluid. It communicates with the middle ear with which it is continuous.

It is composed of the following parts:

- **vestibule**
- **semicircular canals**
- **cochlea**

Vestibule

This forms the entrance to the inner ear and here the oval and round windows are situated, communicating with the middle ear.

Semi-circular canals

These contain specialised structures which, upon movement of the fluid within the membranes, stimulate nerve endings which convey information concerning position of the head and position in space to the brain.

Disease within these structures can cause giddiness (**vertigo**) and loss of balance.

Cochlea

This structure, within the membranous labyrinth, contains the **organ of Corti**, the true organ of hearing. It is coiled like a snail around a tiny bone.

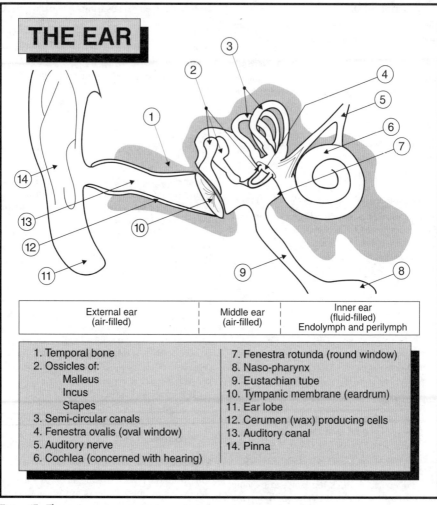

THE EAR

External ear (air-filled)	Middle ear (air-filled)	Inner ear (fluid-filled) Endolymph and perilymph

1. Temporal bone
2. Ossicles of:
   Malleus
   Incus
   Stapes
3. Semi-circular canals
4. Fenestra ovalis (oval window)
5. Auditory nerve
6. Cochlea (concerned with hearing)
7. Fenestra rotunda (round window)
8. Naso-pharynx
9. Eustachian tube
10. Tympanic membrane (eardrum)
11. Ear lobe
12. Cerumen (wax) producing cells
13. Auditory canal
14. Pinna

Figure 47 - The ear.

Within it are numerous specialised nerve endings which convey the effect of sound waves received along the **auditory nerve** for interpretation by the **temporal lobe** of the brain (cerebrum).

Interpretation of sound

The round window bulges outwards as vibration is conducted through the oval window from the stapes, so maintaining the correct pressure of the fluid in the inner ear. In blast injuries these windows may perforate. Sensations of volume, pitch and harmony are perceived due to fluctuations in pressure.

THE NOSE

The sense of smell is received by specialised nerve fibres in the mucous membrane of the nasal cavities and is conveyed to the brain via the **olfactory nerve** for interpretation (see Figure 48).

THE TONGUE

This muscular organ, attached to the **hyoid** bone, contains the **taste buds** and special **receptor cells** which convey the sense of taste (salt, bitter, sweet and sour) to the brain for interpretation. These are found within specialised structures known as **papillae** (see Figure 49).

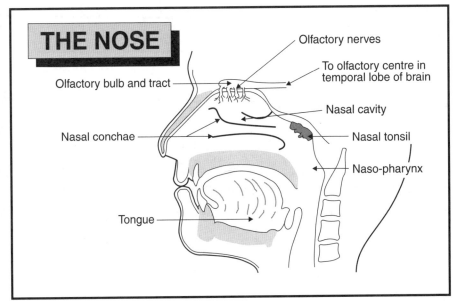

THE NOSE

Olfactory nerves

To olfactory centre in temporal lobe of brain

Olfactory bulb and tract

Nasal cavity

Nasal conchae

Nasal tonsil

Naso-pharynx

Tongue

Figure 48 - The nose.

Other flavours are appreciated in conjunction with the sense of smell. It is for this reason that the sense of taste is affected when the person is suffering from a cold. For the perception of these sensations, the membranes in which the special cells are situated, must be moist.

Taste buds are also present in the mucous membrane of the **palate** and **pharynx**.

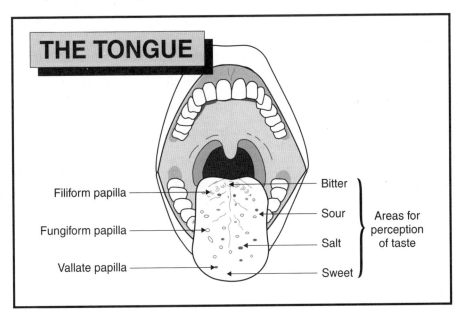

THE TONGUE

Filiform papilla

Bitter

Sour

Areas for perception of taste

Fungiform papilla

Salt

Vallate papilla

Sweet

Figure 49 - The tongue.

ABBREVIATIONS

ABR	auditory brainstem response
Acc	accommodation
AD	right ear (auris dextra)
AS	left ear (auris sinister)
Ast	astigmatism
AU	both ears (aures unitas) or each ear
D	diopter (lens strength)
db	decibel (measurement of sound)
ENT	ear, nose and throat
EOM	extraocular movement
HM	hand movement
IOFB	intraocular foreign body
IOP	intraocular pressure
L&D	light and dark perceived
LCS	left convergent squint (eye turns inwards)
LDS	left divergent squint (eye turns outwards)
OD	oculus dexter (right eye)
OS	oculus sinister (left eye)
OU	oculus uterque (each eye)
PERLA (PERRLA)	pupils equal (round), react to light and accommodation
PND	post-nasal drip (catarrh dripping down the back of the throat from the nasal passages and sinuses)
RCS	right convergent squint (eye turns out-wards)
RDS	right divergent squint (eye turns inwards)
REM	rapid eye movement
SC	without correction (spectacles)
Ts & As	tonsillectomy and adenoidectomy
T+	increased intraocular pressure
T-	decreased intraocular pressure
VA	visual acuity (clarity or accuracy of vision)
VF	visual field

TERMINOLOGY

Blephar/o	eyelid
Cor, core/o	pupil
Irid/o	stem for iris (of eye).
Kerat/o	stem for cornea.
Dacry/o	} stems for tear.
Lachrym/o	
Lacrim/o	
Lacrym/o	
Ocul/o and	stems for eye.
Ophthalm/o	
Opt/o	stem for vision.
Ot/o and Aur/i	stems for ear.
Phak/o	stem for eye lens.
Retin/o	retina
Tympan/o and	stems for ear drum.
Myring/o	
Uve/o	stem for uveal tract.
Blind spot	area of no vision due to optic disc area where there are no sensory visual receptors.
Fovea	see Macula.
Fundus of eye	the whole of area at the back of the eye opposite the pupil.
Macula (fovea)	area on the retina with the greatest number of receptors for sight (central vision).
Ophthalmic optician	person qualified to examine eyes, and prescribe and dispense spectacles.
Ophthalmologist	specialist in the diseases of the eye.
Ophthalmology	scientific study of the eye.
Optician	person who makes and fits spectacles.
Optometrist	person who measures/tests eyes and fits spectacles.
Orthoptist	therapist who treats squints.
Otologist	medical specialist in treating ear disease.
Otology	study of ear disease.
Otorhinolaryngologist	medical specialist in ear, nose and throat disease.

Otorhinolaryngology	study of the ear, nose and throat.
Refraction	bending of light rays to measure the focusing of the eye mechanisms.

DISEASES AND DISORDERS

6/6 vision	the normal ability to be able to read line six of the Snellen chart at six metres.
Amblyopia	dimness of vision.
Aphakia	condition where there is no lens present, e.g. after removal of cataract.
Astigmatism	eye defect usually of shape of cornea which is irregular in curvature, causing blurring of vision.
Aural polyp	pedunculated (stalk-like) tumour in the ear - not malignant.
Blepharitis	inflammation of the eyelids.
Cataract	an opacity of the lens or its capsule causing blurring of sight.
Cauliflower ear	enlargement/deformity of the external ear due to haematoma formation after injury.
Choroiditis	inflammation of the choroid layer of eyeball.
Conduction deafness	loss of hearing due to the failure of the vibrations caused by sound waves to be conducted to specialised nerve cells of the inner ear.
Conjunctivitis	inflammation of the conjunctiva membrane covering eyeball and lining eyelids.
Corneal ulcer	open sore on cornea.
Dacryocystectomy	surgical removal of a tear sac.
Dacryocystitis	inflammation of the tear sacs.
Dacryolith	stone in the tear duct.
Dacryostenosis	narrowing of tear duct.

Dendritic ulcer	corneal ulcer that has tree-like branches in shape (caused by the herpes simplex virus - cold sore).
Ectropion	eversion of eyelid (outward).
Entropion	inversion of the eyelid (inward).
Exophthalmos	abnormal protrusion of the eye.
Glaucoma	a condition where intraocular pressure is raised, which in turn causes damage to the retina leading to blindness if not controlled.
Glue ear/ serous otitis media	presence of catarrh (fluid/pus) in middle ear.
Hemianopia	partial blindness - ability to see only half the visual field.
Hordeolum	'stye' - infection of the eyelash follicle.
Hypermetropia	long-sightedness.
Intraocular pressure	pressure within the eyeball.
Iridocyclitis	inflammation of the iris and ciliary body (from where the lens is suspended).
Iritis	inflammation of the muscular iris of the eye.
Keratitis	inflammation of the cornea.
Labyrinthitis	inflammation of the inner ear.
Macular degeneration	a degeneration of vision due to changes to the macular area of the eye (see Figure 45) which is responsible for maximum vision. At present there is little effective treatment.
Mastoiditis	inflammation of the mastoid antrum (cavity containing porous sieve-like bone) of the temporal bone of the skull.

Meibomian cyst	blockage of ducts of specialised sebaceous glands of the eyelid known as meibomian glands.
Ménières disease	a syndrome causing vertigo (dizziness), tinnitus and deafness.
Myopia	short-sightedness.
Myringitis	inflammation of the eardrum.
Nerve deafness	loss of hearing due to damage or disease of the nerve fibres.
Optic disc	area at the back of the eyeball where there are no rods or cones, and where the optic nerve enters the eyeball - examined with an ophthalmo-scope to detect swelling or abnormali-ty to blood vessels or nervous system.
Otalgia	earache.
Otitis externa	inflammation of the external ear.
Otitis media	inflammation of the middle ear.
Otorrhoea	discharge from the ear.
Otosclerosis	progressive hardening of the membranous bony labyrinth (lining of inner ear); heredi-tary in females - otoliths in middle ear also become fixed so cannot vibrate.
Papilloedema	oedema (free fluid pre-sent) of the optic disc.
Presbyopia	(old sight) long-sight-edness due to failure of the lens capsule to accommodate, i.e. change shape of lens in order to focus close up objects - lens capsule becomes less elastic with the process of ageing.
Proptosis	eyeballs protrude outwards/forwards.

Ptosis	drooping of the eyelid.
Retinal detachment	detachment of the retinal layer of eyeball from the choroid.
Retinitis	inflammation of the retina (nerve layer of the eyeball).
Retinopathy	disease of the retina.
Rodent ulcer	slow growing malignant tumour of the top layer of skin causing destruction of tissue.
Scleritis	inflammation of the sclera (tough outer coat of eyeball).
Scotoma	normal and abnormal 'blind spots' in the visual fields.
Strabismus	squint, i.e. failure of eyes to work evenly together.
Uveitis	inflammation of the uveal tract (iris, choroid and ciliary body).

PROCEDURES AND EQUIPMENT

Audiogram	the recorded mea-surement of hearing.
Audiometer	instrument used to measure hearing.
Audiometry	measurement of hearing.
Auriscope (otoscope)	lighted instrument used to examine ear canal and eardrum.
Corneal graft	grafting a donor cornea into place.
Cryosurgery	cooling or freezing the area which is being operated upon.
Decibels	a unit of hearing (mea-surement of sound).
Ear syringing	removal of excessive wax by syringing exter-nal auditory canal with warm water.
Enucleation	removal of an organ from its place, e.g. eyeball from socket.
Grommets	special valves fitted into eardrum to

release pressure in middle ear and drain fluid.

Iridectomy surgical removal of portion of iris, forming an artificial 'hole'.

Laser surgery surgery using a laser beam instead of scalpel or stitching.

Miotics drops which constrict the pupil of the eye.

Mydriatics drops used to dilate the pupil of the eye.

Myringotomy cutting into the eardrum.

Ophthalmoscope a lighted instrument used to examine the interior of the eyeball.

Otoscope instrument for examining the ear (see Auriscope).

Otoscopy examination of the ear with a lighted instrument.

Paracentesis tympani drawing off of fluid within the middle ear.

Perimetry plotting of the visual fields.

Radical mastoidectomy removal of large area of mastoid bone area to prevent further infection and drain area of pus (common before advent of antibiotics), a complication of otitis media.

Removal of cataract operation to remove the opaque lens.

Rinne's Test test for deafness using a tuning fork placed on the auditory opening of the ear. When the patient ceases to hear the ringing tone it is placed on the bony area below, known as the mastoid process. In normal hearing it will not be heard at this point, but in conditions of middle ear deafness a tone will still be heard by the patient.

Slit lamp special machine used to examine the eyes.

Snellen chart chart used to test visual acuity, i.e. sight.

Stapedectomy surgical removal of the stapes (stirrup bone) of the middle ear.

Tarsoplasty reshaping of the eyelid.

Tonometer an instrument used to measure intra-ocular pressure (within the eyeball).

Trephine instrument used for cutting away a circle of tissue.

Tympanoplasty reshaping the eardrum.

Visual acuity the acuteness of sight.

Visual fields measurement or plotting of the area of vision (perimetry) to establish any damage (blind spot will be normal area).

Weber's test test for comparison of the bone conduction of hearing in both ears. A tuning fork is struck and placed on the vertex of the skull. The patient indicates in which ear it is heard the loudest. In conditions of middle ear deafness it is louder in the affected ear.

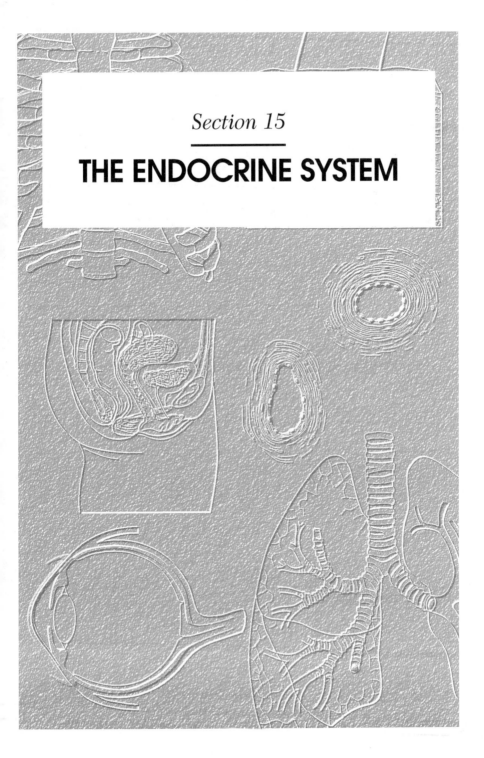

Section 15

THE ENDOCRINE SYSTEM

FUNCTION

This is the system concerned with the production of chemical messengers (**hormones**) which are secreted from a ductless gland (**endocrine gland**) directly into the blood stream to activate a target organ (see Figure 50).

STRUCTURE

The endocrine system consists of the following:

- **Pituitary gland**
- **Adrenal glands**
- **Thyroid gland**
- **Parathyroid glands**
- **Pancreas**
- **Ovaries**
- **Testes**
- **Thymus**
- **Pineal body**

Pituitary gland

This is situated at the base of the brain and is the size of a pea. It is known as the master gland or 'leader of the endocrine orchestra' because it controls many of the other endocrine glands. It has an **anterior** and **posterior** lobe which produce many hormones (see Figure 51). It is controlled by the **hypothalamus** of the brain, situated immediately above.

Anterior lobe

This produces the following hormones:

Adrenocorticotrophic hormone (ACTH)	stimulates adrenal gland cortex to produce corticosteroids and sex hormones.
Growth hormone (GH)	stimulates growth of bone especially long bones.

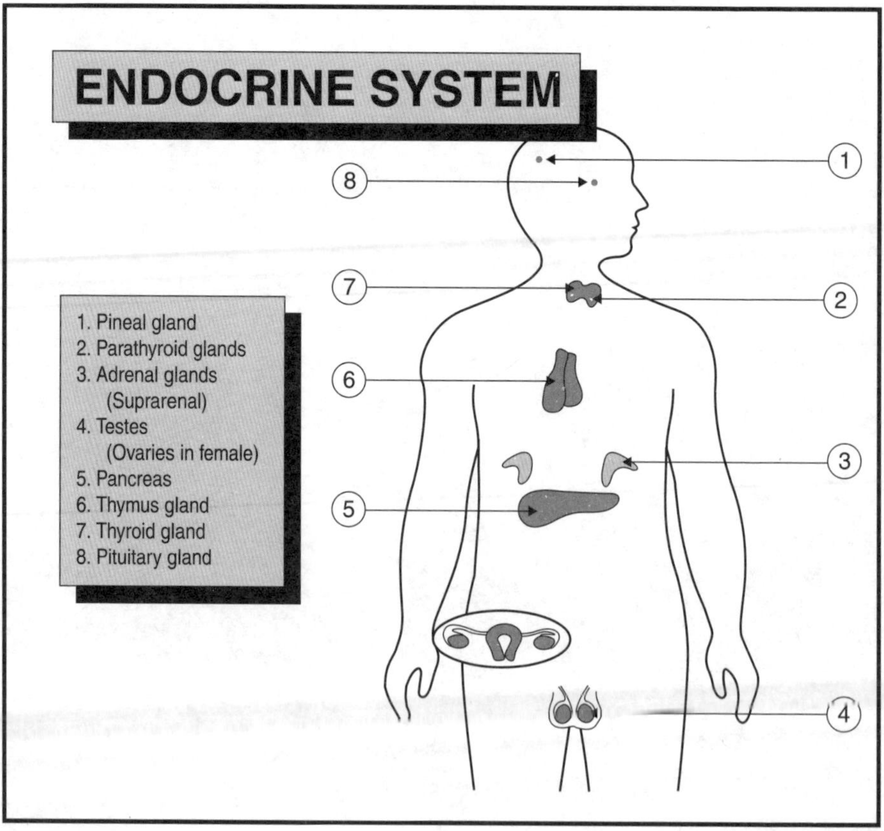

ENDOCRINE SYSTEM

1. Pineal gland
2. Parathyroid glands
3. Adrenal glands (Suprarenal)
4. Testes (Ovaries in female)
5. Pancreas
6. Thymus gland
7. Thyroid gland
8. Pituitary gland

Figure 50 - The endocrine system.

Thyroid stimulating hormone (TSH)	stimulates **thyroid gland** to produce **thyroxin**.
Melanin stimulating hormone (MSH)	produces pigmentation of skin but is normally inhibited by action of adrenal cortex hormones.
Gonadotrophic hormones (FSH & LH)	Follicle stimulating hormone (FSH) stimulates the follicles of ovaries causing egg (ovum) to ripen ready for release. In males it stimulates the testes.
Prolactin or luteotrophic hormone (LTH)	stimulates production of milk.

Growth hormone (GH) affects the growth of long bones. A deficiency will cause stunted growth or **dwarfism** in children. Excess will cause **gigantism**, while in adults, whose long bones can no longer grow, it will cause enlargement of flat bones of the face, hands and feet (**acromegaly**).

The other hormones mentioned act upon target organs, which are influenced in the production of their own hormones. These include the **ovaries**, **testes**, **thyroid** and **adrenal** function. The production of milk by the breast is stimulated by **prolactin**.

Posterior lobe

This produces:

- **Oxytocin**
- **Pitressin** or **vasopressin**

Oxytocin affects the contraction of the smooth muscle of the uterus in pregnancy and childbirth, and the ejection of milk from the breast in suckling.

Pitressin, also known as **antidiuretic hormone (ADH)**, stimulates the tubules of the kidney to reabsorb water and mineral salts, keeping the correct balance in the body. Absence of ADH produces a disease known as **diabetes insipidus**, where copious dilute urine is produced.

Adrenal glands

The adrenal glands (**suprarenal glands**), situated on the top of each kidney, are composed of two parts - an outside portion (**cortex**) and a middle (**medulla**) which produce different secretions and are stimulated by the pituitary gland.

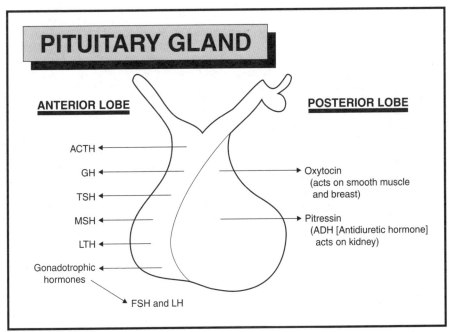

Figure 51 - The pituitary gland.

123

Cortex

The cortex produces **steroids** which affect salt balance, protein and glucose metabolism, growth and muscle tone. Sex hormones are also produced.

In deficiency of these hormones, the patient suffers from **Addison's disease** and is administered **cortisone**. Excess produces **Cushing's syndrome**.

Medulla

The medulla produces **adrenaline**, the stress hormone concerned with preparation of the body for the 'fight or flight' mechanism, whereby heart rate and respirations quicken, energy is released by the liver and muscles, and the body can respond to fear and excitement.

Thyroid gland

This gland is stimulated by the **pituitary gland**. It is situated in the neck, in front of the larynx and is concerned with the basic **metabolism** of the body. It produces a hormone called **thyroxine** which requires iodine in the diet for its production. **Iodine** is added to salt used for cooking purposes for this reason.

Excessive secretion causes **hyperthyroidism** or **thyrotoxicosis** with increased heart rate, excessive energy, nervousness, protruding eyeballs etc. Treatment is usually surgical and a **partial thyroidectomy** is performed.

Under-secretion, or **hyposecretion**, causes a disease known as **myxoedema** where the patient is mentally and physically slow and all body functions are sluggish as metabolism is at a minimal rate. Treatment is with thyroxine and the effect can be miraculous as the patient returns to normal.

In childhood, deficiency produces **cretinism** and this is routinely tested (screened) for at birth.

Parathyroid glands

Deep within the thyroid gland lie the parathyroids. These produce **parathyroid hormone** (**PTH**), which is involved in the control of **calcium metabolism** and the level of calcium in the bloodstream and in the bone.

Pancreas

The endocrine function of the pancreas, situated in the abdominal cavity close to the stomach, is the control of **carbohydrate metabolism** in the body.

Insulin is produced directly into the bloodstream from special cells known as the 'islets of Langerhans'. These regulate the levels of glucose in the blood and allow conversion of sugars to glucose for storage in the liver and muscles, ready for release when required.

Deficiency of insulin causes a condition known as **diabetes mellitus**, which may be treated with insulin injections. Insulin cannot be taken by mouth as it is destroyed by the gastric secretions of the stomach.

Ovaries and testes

These are the **gonads** (produce the sex cells). Their role in hormone secretion is to produce **oestrogens** and **progesterone** in the female and **androgens** in the male, the main one being **testosterone**. They are stimulated by the pituitary gland.

Thymus

This is situated in the chest (thoracic) cavity near the trachea upon the major blood vessels. It is important in childhood and puberty for growth and development. It is concerned with the production of **lymphoid tissue**, **lymphocytes** and **immunity**.

Pineal body

This is a structure within the **cerebrum** of the brain which was probably a vestigial third eye (remains from animal development). Its endocrine function is not clear, but it may have effects upon 'diurnal rhythm' ('body clock') and production of sex hormones.

ABBREVIATIONS

ACTH	adrenocorticotrophic hormone
ADH	antidiuretic hormone (pitressin)
FBS	fasting blood sugar
FSH	follicle stimulating hormone
GH	growth hormone
IDDM	insulin-dependent diabetes mellitus
LH	luteinising hormone
LTH	luteotrophic hormone (prolactin)
MSH	melanin stimulating hormone
NIDDM	non-insulin-dependent diabetes mellitus

PBI	protein-bound iodine
PTH	parathyroid hormone
RAI	radioactive iodine
RAIU	radioactive iodine uptake
T$_3$	triiodothyronine (thyroid hormone)
T$_4$	thyroxine (thyroid hormone)
TSH	thyroid stimulating hormone

TERMINOLOGY

Aden/o	stem for gland.
Adren/o	stem for adrenal gland
Cortic/o	stem referring to the cortex (outer portion) of an organ.
Endocrin/o	endocrine (concerning hormones)
Parathyr/o	stem for parathyroid gland.
Hypophys/o	pituitary gland
Medull/o	medulla (middle/inside portion)
Thym/o	thymus gland
Thyr/o	stem for thyroid gland.
Basal metabolic rate (BMR)	the rate at which the body cells work in using food substances and oxygen to create energy and waste products of carbon dioxide (CO_2) and water (H_2O) - measured at complete rest.
Pitressin (vasopressin)	antidiuretic hormone (ADH) increases reabsorption by the kidney tubules to prevent dehydration (water loss by the body).

DISEASES AND DISORDERS

Acromegaly	overgrowth of flat bones of face, hands and feet caused by excessive growth hormone in adults.
Addison's disease	insufficient adrenal cortex hormones produced causing weakness, pigmentation of skin, wasting etc.
Cretinism	under-secretion of thyroxine hormone in babies - present at birth (congenital) causing mental and physical retardation.
Cushing's syndrome	excessive adrenal cortex hormones (steroids) causing abnormal distribution of hair, fat and shrinking (atrophy) of genitals.
Diabetes insipidus	deficiency of pitressin hormone resulting in copious amounts of urine being produced.
Dwarfism	insufficient growth hormone produced causing lack of growth of long bones in children.
Exophthalmos	abnormal protrusion of the eyeball.
Gigantism	excessive growth hormone in children, causes excessive growth of long bones.
Goitre	
Simple goitre	enlargement of the thyroid gland in the neck - can cause pressure upon the trachea embarrassing breathing. Enlargement of the thyroid gland due to lack of iodine in the diet, also known as 'Derbyshire neck' as there is no iodine in Derbyshire water.
Malignant goitre	enlargement of thyroid gland due to hyperthyroidism causing severe toxic symptoms which are dangerous to health.
Hyperparathyroidism	excessive production of parathyroid hormone (PTH) from

parathyroid glands - causes excessive
calcium in the blood and can cause deposits of
calcium salts (stones) in the kidneys.

Hypersecretion oversecretion.

Hypoparathyroidism insufficient production
of hormone PTH from
parathyroid glands
causing insufficient
calcium in the blood.

Hyposecretion undersecretion.

Myxoedema undersecretion of
thyroxine hormone in
adults causing slowed
metabolism, mental
and physical dull-
ness, loss of eye-
brows and hair,
oedema (free fluid)
of the face, etc.

Osteitis fibrosis cystica formation of cysts in
the bone due to
excess parathyroid
hormone production,
calcium salts are
removed from the
bones into the blood.

Tetany involuntary spasms of
the muscles, particu-
larly of the hands and
feet, caused by low
levels of calcium in
the blood.

Thyrotoxicosis hyperthyroidism -
oversecretion of the
hormone thyroxine,
causing raised pulse,
tremor, bulging eyes
(exophthalmos), loss
of weight, enlarge-
ment of thyroid
gland etc.

PROCEDURES AND EQUIPMENT

Hypophysectomy surgical removal of
the pituitary gland (or
partial removal).

Thyroidectomy partial or complete
surgical removal of
the thyroid gland.

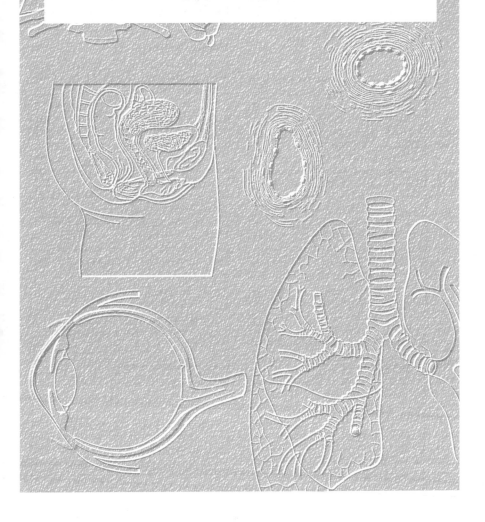

THE X-RAY DEPARTMENT AND ITS SERVICES

This hospital department is primarily concerned with the diagnosis and investigation of disease using **X-rays** (ionising rays). It is also involved with newer types of investigations such as **ultrasound**, and **magnetic resonance imaging** (**MRI**). In hospitals which do not have a separate **nuclear medicine department**, diagnostic techniques which use radioactive isotopes are performed in the X-ray department. Therapy involving the use of **radioactive isotopes**, and **radiotherapy** used in the treatment of cancer, may also form part of the work of this department.

The diagnostic **radiologist** is the medical doctor who specialises in this field, while diagnostic **radiographers** are the professional staff involved in the many procedures. Where such staff are involved in treatment of disease they are known as therapeutic radiologists and ragiographers.

X-RAYS

X-rays, also known as **Röentgen rays**, are short waves which are potentially very harmful, unless carefully controlled, and extreme precautions are enforced to ensure safety to both patients and staff. Scatter of the rays from the X-ray table will occur as the pictures are taken.

Careful technical design, regular testing of machines and stringent training of all staff are employed to this effect. Monitoring of exposure to the radiation by staff, is measured by a special type of counter attached to the person's clothing. The wearing, by the radiographers and other personnel involved in procedures, of lead aprons, through which X-rays will not penetrate, is essential for their protection. Children and pregnant women are given a shield of lead material to prevent the ovaries or testes, containing immature ova and sperm, becoming affected by the radiation. X-rays of pregnant women are only performed when absolutely essential, to avoid potential damage to the fetus.

Genetic damage

While all cells are sensitive to radiation, dividing or immature cells are even more vulnerable and damage to the genetic material can occur.

Whenever possible, routine X-ray investigations are avoided during the latter part of the menstrual cycle, when a woman of childbearing age could have conceived. It is for this reason that a section for LMP (last menstrual period) is to be found on X-ray request forms.

DIAGNOSTIC RADIOLOGY

This is the term used when X-rays are used for diagnosis.

Medical imaging

X-rays are able to pass through skin and soft tissue. They can then act upon certain photographic chemicals to produce a permanent record known as a **radiograph**. They also have the property of being able to 'light up' a **fluorescent screen**, so producing a visible image of body organs on the screen, which can then be transferred to a TV monitor.

Preparation of the patient

Some X-ray investigations require special preparation of the patient by fasting, giving of laxatives or other special requirements.

Simple straight X-rays

X-rays will penetrate different types of tissue at different intensities, according to the thickness and density of the body structures through which they are passing. They are reflected by bone tissue containing calcium salts, i.e. the latter are **opaque** to X-rays. Soft tissues will appear more transparant than bone, which will appear as dense opaque structures; air present in the lungs and abdomen will give a completely transparant appearance on an X-ray film or **radiograph**. In **simple straight X-rays**, only a certain amount of information will be obtained from the varying degree of shadow produced. These pictures are taken on a special film and developed by the dark room technician for later reading and report by the radiologist.

Examples:

Investigations for:
- **fractured bones**,
- **pneumonia**,
- swallowed **foreign bodies** (e.g. safety pins).

Image enhancement

However, with the use of modern techniques, the scope of investigation of the body by X-ray has been transformed. The investigation of soft tissues requires lower radiation doses which will travel more slowly through the differing densities of tissues producing varying degrees of shadow. This differentiation of soft tissue to a higher resolution is also enhanced by implementation of techniques such as the application of the photographic process (**xeroradiography**), by use of specially sensitised film (as in the process of **mammography**) and **computer-enhanced imaging** techniques (as in **CAT** (**CT**) **scanning**) allowing the clear demonstration of **lesions** (abnormal changes). These techniques are now widely used in diagnostic procedures.

Fluoroscopy

This procedure is used for live visual examination of the patient by the radiologist; the image appears upon a fluorescent screen or monitor. This technique is particularly useful for examining movements such as **swallowing** and the propulsion of food along the alimentary canal by **peristalsis**. Pictures are also taken for later inspection by the radiologist. **Contrast medium** is usually used in these investigations, which include those of the urinary tract, gastrointestinal tract and blood vessels.

Contrast medium

The introduction of a '**contrast medium**' or **radio-opaque** substance (a substance which will absorbs X-rays) allows blood vessels and hollow organs to be clearly demonstrated. Substances, such as **barium sulphate** and radio-opaque **iodine dyes**, are used either by swallowing (ingestion) or via injection.

Examples:
Investigation for gastric ulcer etc. by **barium meal**, **barium enema** for tumours of the bowel.
Intravenous pyelogram (IVP) for introduction of radio-opaque iodine to show kidneys and bladder.
Air may also be used as a contrast medium when injected into a structure which normally absorbs X-rays. As the air will absorb considerably less X-radiation, it is said to be **radio-translucent** and will give a transparant effect on the screen or film.

Examples:
Introduction of air in a **ventriculogram** for investigation of the brain.

Examples of organ imaging

The following are examples of special procedures performed in organ imaging investigations:

Mammography

This special X-ray procedure involves the compression of the breast tissue between plastic plates which, together with low density X-rays,

allows enhanced imaging of the soft tissues. Special film plate and processing are also used. It is now widely used in the detection of cancerous lesions before any clinical signs or symptoms are apparent (see Section 20).

Thermography

This is a method which records the emission of infrared radiation or heat rays from the body. Actively dividing cells produce more heat than other less active cells and show 'hot' spots in a picture. Inflammation of tissue will also have this effect.

Examples:
Investigation and monitoring of arthritis.

CAT or CT scan (computerised axial tomography or computerised tomography)

This is a method whereby the tissue density of any part of the head and trunk is examined by X-rays in minute layered sections. The whole process is computerised to produce numerous pictures which are used to detect any abnormality. A **radio-opaque** substance may also be injected during the procedure to give further information to aid diagnosis.

Examples:
Investigation for tumours of the central nervous system etc.

MRI (magnetic resonance imaging)

This is a procedure which is mainly used to investigate the **central nervous system**. Powerful magnets are used to activate the hydrogen component of body cells. Sensitive detectors reflect this activity, which is then translated into high resolution images by a computerised system.

As this procedure does not involve the use of X-rays, there is less risk to the patient than with CAT (CT) scanning. It will also detect smaller abnormalities.

Examples:
Investigation of neurological conditions, e.g. multiple sclerosis.

PET – Positron Emission Tomography

This type of scan demonstrates the **functioning** of cells. With the use of an isotope it shows visually oxygen uptake, blood flow and glucose metabolism of specific areas of the body.

Nuclear medicine

This method of investigation uses **radio-isotopes**, i.e. unstable compounds which give off radiation.

These substances are introduced into the body, usually orally or by injection.

Because different tissues absorb chemicals at different rates, specific organs can be investigated using this method. A special detector picks up the radiation being given off from the area where it has been absorbed and converts it into a coloured picture.

Bone scan or scintigram

This is used to detect bone cancer at a very early stage; cancerous bone cells absorb more of the isotope than normal bone cells and so a brighter, or 'hotter', area is produced on the picture.

Ultrasonic scan

The ultrasound department is found within the X-ray department of many hospitals, although sometimes it is part of the obstetric department.

Ultrasound is a term used to describe high frequency vibration beyond the audible range, known as **ultrasonic waves**. 'Echoes' are reflected backwards when a beam of ultrasonic sounds is made to travel through the body tissues. Images are produced on a television-type screen which give information concerning position, size and shape of the body structures. There are two types of scanning, type A and type B, each of which gives a different range of imaging. As ultrasound does not involve the use of X-rays, it is a safer procedure for the patient.

Examples:
Investigation of fetal development/prostatic enlargement etc.

Doppler system

This is a type of ultrasonic scanning which produces audible signals and records movement within the body.

Examples:
Investigation of blood flow in blood vessels, e.g. for diagnosis of **DVT** (deep vein thrombosis)/heart movements.

USE OF X-RAYS AS THERAPY

This is usually part of the department of nuclear medicine. The doctor in charge of this department is a **radiotherapist**.

Radio-isotopes, usually of **radium** or **cobalt**, are used to treat conditions such as cancerous tumours. Cancerous cells are, by their nature, immature, rapidly dividing cells and are more susceptible to exposure by radiation than normal cells. This is the principle of radiation treatment.

Normal dividing cells, such as blood cells, are also damaged by the treatment, which is why anaemia and lowered immunity can be side-effects of the treatment.

Carefully controlled dosages are given, measured for each individual patient. Great care must be taken of the skin surrounding the target area, which must be kept dry throughout and after treatment to avoid breakdown of the tissue.

X-RAY REQUESTS

Special request forms for X-ray procedures are completed with the details of the patient and the type of X-ray required. **It is important that all details are correct, including the information concerning the LMP (last menstrual period).**

After the radiologist at the hospital has reported on the results of the investigation, copies are despatched to the doctor/GP who requested the procedure.

Costing for X-rays is divided into various categories, according to the complexity of the procedures.

ABBREVIATIONS

AP&L	anterior, posterior and lateral
IVP	intravenous pyelogram
IVU	intravenous urogram
PET	positron emission tomography
RP	retrograde pyelogram

(See also abbreviations in other specialities)

TERMINOLOGY

Angiogram (-ography)	X-ray investigation of blood vessels using an opaque medium.
Aortogram (-ography)	1. recording of pulse in graph form 2. demonstration of aorta using opaque medium.
Barium X-ray	X-ray using barium sulphate as contrast medium to demonstrate any abnormality in the digestive tract.
Meal	the stomach and small intestine.
Swallow	the oesophagus.

Enema	the large intestine.
Follow through	the whole tract.
Bronchogram (-ography)	X-ray examination of bronchi and bronchioles using an opaque medium.
Cephalopelvimetry	measurement of fetal head in relation to maternal pelvis
Cholangiogram (-ography)	X-ray examination of the ducts of the gallbladder using an opaque medium.
Cholecystogram (-ography)	X-ray examination of the gallbladder using an opaque medium given by mouth.
Encephalogram (-ography)	X-ray of the brain by insertion of air.
Hysterosalpingogram (-ography)	X-ray of uterus and fallopian tubes using an opaque medium to detect blockage or abnormality.
Intravenous pyelogram (-ography)	X-ray of the kidney and its pelvis after injection of an opaque medium.
Intravenous urogram (-ography)	X-ray of urinary tract highlighting bladder after injecting opaque medium.
Mammogram (-ography)	special X-ray of the breast to detect early cancer.
Micturating cystogram	X-ray of the bladder for investigation of stress incontinence etc.
Myelogram	X-ray of spinal cord using a radio-opaque dye.
Nuclear medicine	the use of radio-active isotopes in diagnosis and treatment of disease.

Radiculogram	X-ray of spinal cord using radio-opaque dye which highlights the roots of the lumbar-sacral spinal nerves.
Radiographer	a professional person qualified in: 1. technical use of X-rays (diagnostic). 2. applying treatment with radiation (therapeutic).
Radiologist	medical specialist concerned with radiation and X-rays.
Radiology	scientific study of radiation and its effects.
Radiotherapy	the use of radiation to treat disease.
Retrograde cholangio-pancreotography	special X-ray examination of the bile and pancreatic ducts by insertion of a radio-opaque dye via an endoscope.
Retrograde pyelogram (-ography)	X-ray of ureters, bladder and pelvis of kidney by insertion of an opaque dye via catheters in the ureters from the urethra below.
Sialogram (-ography)	X-ray of salivary glands using an opaque medium.
Splenangiogram	X-ray of spleen and vessels using an opaque medium.
Splenogram	X-ray of spleen using an opaque medium.
Ventriculogram	X-ray of the ventricles of brain by insertion of air.

N.B. for other types of investigations see various specialities.

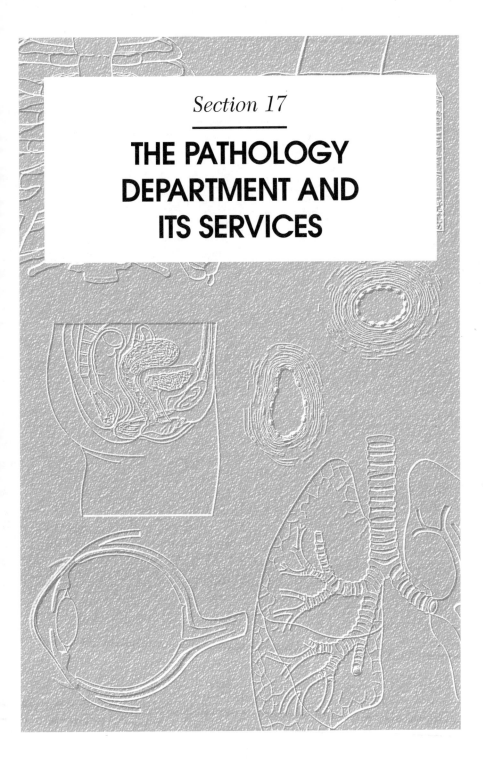

Section 17

THE PATHOLOGY DEPARTMENT AND ITS SERVICES

This hospital department is involved in special tests concerning various samples from the living body used to assist in the diagnosis and prognosis of disease. The mortuary is also part of the pathology department and post-mortems are performed by the pathologist, who is also the specialist doctor in charge of the whole department. Recently, with the advent of fundholding in general practice, private laboratories have been involved with providing services.

ORGANISATION

As previously mentioned, apart from the chief pathologist, there will be the following personnel employed in the department:

- **Pathologists** (doctors) dependent on size of hospital
- **Scientific officers**
- **Trainees**
- **Laboratory assistants**
- **Phlebotomists** (staff who take blood from patients)
- **Administrative** and **clerical** staff
- **Morticians**
- **Porters**

SAFETY

Stringent health and safety precautions must be observed in this department as in any other hospital area. The risk is immense as the specimens handled are hazardous due to their disease-producing potential.

SECTIONS

The following sections are part of the laboratory:

- **Haematology** (including **serology**)
- **Biochemistry** or **clinical chemistry**
- **Cytology**
- **Histology** or **histopathology** (including **oncology**)
- **Microbiology**
- **Virology**
- **Epidemiology**

The Public Health Laboratory is usually part of the pathology department, sharing facilities. This is involved in routine checking of food, milk and water samples, as well as being involved in the control of infectious diseases. Suspected carriers of infection are screened and samples from them are tested in this laboratory.

Haematology

This is one of the largest sections of the laboratory and is sometimes connected with the work of the **Regional Blood Transfusion Centre** where blood for donation is stored. Any blood ready for transfusion will be kept here in a special refrigerated unit. **Dried plasma** ready for use will also be available for emergencies.

The areas within the department will include those investigating blood cells, and the **serology section** involved with investigations on the serum of blood.

Tests

Various tests will be performed on cells and serum sent from the hospital and general practice in the various containers required, e.g. **haemoglobin estimation**. The department's phlebotomists also collect blood from patients attending for this purpose.

Biochemistry

This section is involved in investigation of the chemical content of the blood, urine or other body fluid.

Tests

As well as routine tests for electrolytes, hormones etc, samples from patients suffering from drug overdose are analysed here.

Cytology

This section examines cells to detect any abnormality.

Tests

These include cervical cells present in **cervical smears**, as well as cells from the respiratory tract and other areas under investigation. The aim, in many cases, is to detect early abnormalities (precancerous conditions) in order to prevent the development of a cancerous condition.

Histology or histopathology

This section is involved in preparing sections of tissue which have been removed from the living patient at a **biopsy**.

Tests

These tissue sections are then examined under the microscope to diagnose and classify any abnormality, such as cancer.

Oncology

This section, often part of the histology department, examines cells from tumours.

Tests

These involve microscopic examination of sections of suspected malignant tumours from any area of the body.

Microbiology

This section is involved in investigation of samples taken from wounds and other areas to detect microscopic organisms which are causing disease.

Classification of micro-organisms

The main ones are:

bacteria	e.g. staphylococcus
viruses	e.g. measles virus (Morbilli)
fungi	e.g. thrush (Candida albicans)
protozoa	e.g. amoeba

Tests

These include those on urine, sputum and blood samples etc, from which the organisms are cultured, i.e. put into or onto a **medium** which allows the organism to grow.

Culture

The **culture plate**, or other medium, impregnated with the specimen, is placed in an **incubator** at body temperature and left for any organisms present to multiply. The resulting culture is then removed and stained with special dye. This is taken up by the cells, which enables them to be viewed under the microscope. In this way the organism can be recognised and named.

Agar (from seaweed) is commonly used as culture medium and blood can be added as a nutrient. Not all micro-organisms will grow outside the body. Viruses require living tissue, such as blood or eggs, for culture.

Sensitivity

Bacteria respond to antibiotic treatment, but it is important that the most effective one is used to fight the infection in the patient. The culture plate used contains various areas of specific antibiotics to determine to which of them the organism is **sensitive**. The bacteria will grow around and over those antibiotics to which they have become **resistant**. A space will be left around those to which the organism is sensitive.

Virology

This section is concerned with the isolation and culture of viruses. As with all areas in the laboratory, stringent safety precautions must be taken, but here special **fume cupboards** are used to prevent the spread of any viruses present.

Tests

These are for the isolation and classification of any viruses in the specimens. Only viruses large enough to be filtered can be detected.

Epidemiology

This department, which is concerned with the study of the causes of disease (including social factors), may be attached to the pathology department or be a separate unit. Recently, some epidemiology departments have been involved in the monitoring of extra-contractual referrals of patients (patients referred to a hospital with which the health authority has no contract for services).

COLLECTION OF SPECIMENS

Types of specimen

The following are some of the common specimens sent for investigation:

Wound swabs **Nasal swabs** **Throat swabs**	plain swabs usually placed in nutrient broth after collection to prevent organisms dying.
Urine	MSU (midstream specimen of urine) usually for C&S (culture and sensitivity).
	EMU (early morning urine) usually for pregnancy test.
	CSU (catheter specimen of urine) - if patient has an indwelling catheter - not usually a routine specimen.
Faeces	for culture or content, e.g. fat, usually a series of three specimens.
High vaginal swab (HVS)	charcoal swab often used for culture.
Sputum	for culture or oncology, single or three specimens.
Blood	there are different containers for differing tests. Anti-clotting agents are included in some containers from

laboratories. Tops and labels of bottles are colour-coded.

Histology   tissue placed in pot with preservative (prevents drying out of cells).

Cervical smears   on special named slides. Fixative must be added immediately after collection and allowed to dry, before placing in container (see Figure 52).

Vomit   this may be sent in cases of overdose or poisoning, together with any urine passed.

In hospital, specimens of pleural fluid, cerebrospinal fluid etc. are also taken.

Rules for collection and despatch of specimens

It is most important that all rules are followed concerning pathology specimens. They are classed as a hazard within the COSHH (Control of Substances Hazardous to Health) Regulations in health and safety requirements. If five or more people are employed, general practices and hospitals should have written health and safety policies to protect the safety of their staff, and the handling of specimens should be included.

- Specimens must be clearly identifiable as to the patient and the source; laboratory personnel will not accept specimens which do not comply.

- Gloves should be worn when handling specimens - if a rigid container is kept in

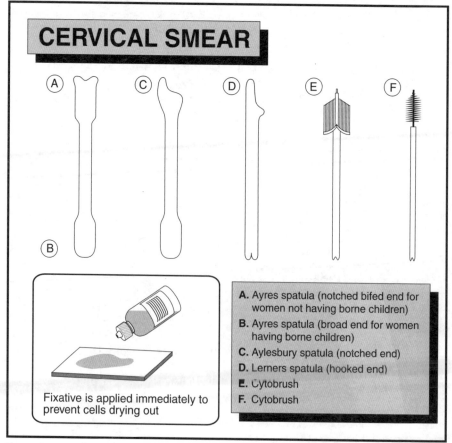

CERVICAL SMEAR

Fixative is applied immediately to prevent cells drying out

A. Ayres spatula (notched bifed end for women not having borne children)
B. Ayres spatula (broad end for women having borne children)
C. Aylesbury spatula (notched end)
D. Lerners spatula (hooked end)
E. Cytobrush
F. Cytobrush

Figure 52 - Cervical smear equipment.

the reception area, patients can be requested to place their specimens in it themselves when bringing them to the surgery. In this way the box can be collected by the practice nurse and the receptionist does not normally need to handle the specimen.

- All forms and labels **must** be correctly completed and legible; clinical details **must** be included.
- All tops must be firmly fixed.
- Specimens (except smears) should remain upright.
- The request form must be placed in the plastic envelope provided and **must not** be in contact with the specimen itself.
- **High-risk specimens** must be labelled with the warning label as well as the form.
- Special care must be taken with common names, e.g. John Smith, and any middle names included.
- Postage of specimens must comply with Post Office regulations concerning **bio-hazards**, which include packaging and labelling requirements. Specimens **must** be sent by **first class** post or **data post**.
- **High-risk specimens must not be posted - whoever posts any specimen is legally liable**.

Patients should be given the following instructions:

- How to collect their own specimen (a leaflet is preferable);
- Where it must be taken and the times of the laboratory;
- How to obtain the results and that an appointment should be made accordingly.

Delay

If there is any delay in the despatch of specimens to the laboratory (apart from cervical smears and histology specimens) they should be placed in the ordinary part of the refrigerator. This should be provided for this purpose and must not be the one used for food. **Never place specimens of blood etc. on a radiator**. Stale specimens can give false results.

PREVENTION OF CROSS-INFECTION

It is important that hands are washed after handling any specimen. Waterproof plasters should always be placed on any broken skin surfaces when working at the surgery.

Blood and body fluids may contain the viruses of hepatitis B, HIV or other pathogens. Needles and other **sharps**, such as scalpel blades, must be placed in the sharp boxes provided, together with used syringes. These are collected and effectively disposed of by incineration to prevent spread of disease. They should never be more than two-thirds full.

There have been incidents of '**needle-stick injuries**' occurring where needles have been placed in the ordinary waste bin and unsuspecting staff have been injured in this way when handling the bag involved. **This can only occur with bad practice by other members of staff.**

Needle-stick injuries

In the event of a 'needle-stick' injury, there are certain rules which must be followed. These events must be **reported immediately** to the named person in the health and safety policy and to the doctor responsible.

Clinical waste

This is also a hazard and includes dressings and linen soiled with body fluid. Special colour-coded bags are used to prevent ordinary disposal or accidental mishandling.

Immunisation

It is recommended that those staff exposed to the risk of hepatitis B infection are offered protection with immunisation. This is given to practice nurses and personnel regularly coming into contact with blood and body fluids. Some GPs offer it to all surgery staff.

REPORTS

Results of tests will be returned to the doctor requesting the investigation. Urgent results may be sent by telephone from the laboratory, but would only usually be given to the doctor directly. The growing use of modems on computers will probably result in direct transmission of results, but the important requirement of **confidentiality** must be ensured. Similarly, this must be maintained in the use of fax machines, where mistakes can so easily be made.

ABBREVIATIONS

This has already been included in the terminology of the blood (Section 4), but a further explanation is included for some of the common tests per-is included for some of the common tests performed in the laboratory.

AHF	antihaemophilic factor VIII
APTT	activated partial thromboplastin time
AST°	aspartate transaminase (cardiac enzyme)
BUN	blood urea nitrogen
C&S	culture and sensitivity
CPK°	creatinine phosphokinase (cardiac enzyme)
ESR	erythrocyte sedimentation rate (rate at which red cells drop to the bottom of the tube) - it is read after one hour, raised in cases of tuberculosis, rheumatic fever and other inflammatory diseases - shows the progress of a disease.
FBC	full blood count - gives the total numbers of all the different blood cells for a comparison with the normal ranges. White cells increase in the presence of infection:

Erythrocytes (red cells)
Leucocytes (white cells) — polymorphonuclear leucocytes:
>> neutrophils
>> basophils
>> eosinophils
non-granular leucocytes:
>> lymphocytes
>> mononocytes

Platelets or thrombocytes (clotting cells)

FBS	fasting blood sugar to determine diabetes mellitus or low blood sugars, performed in early morning before any intake of food
GOT°	glutamiooralo acetic transaminase (cardiac enzyme)
GTT	glucose tolerance test to diagnose diabetes mellitus

Hb	haemoglobin is the iron compound carrying oxygen

Normal levels are:
>*women* 12.5 - 16.0 g/dl (grams per decilitre).
>*men* 14.0 - 18.0 g/dl. The variation in the female is caused by blood loss at menstruation.

HbA₁	blood test for diabetes which shows the amount of glucose that has bound to the haemoglobin of the red cell
HDL	high-density lipoprotein
LD°	lactate dehydrogenase (cardiac enzyme)
LDL	low-density lipoprotein
LFT	liver function test, to diagnose liver disease
MC&S	microscopy culture and sensitivity
MCV	mean corpuscular volume (size of cell)
MRSA	multiple resistant staphylococcus aureus, a resistant strain of bacteria
RBC	red blood cells
T₄	serum thyroxine test for thyroid disease
TPHA	*treponema pallidum* haemagglutination assay (blood test for syphilis)
U&Es	urea and electrolytes; urea is the part of protein broken down by the liver for excretion by the kidneys - raised in kidney damage and dehydration; electrolytes in body fluid include **sodium, potassium, calcium, magnesium, bicarbonates, chlorides** and **phosphates**
VDRL	veneral disease research laboratory (for syphilis)
WBC	white blood count - this is raised in infection, inflammation and

leukaemia, different types according to the type of cause

°These enzymes also show changes in metabolism of other tissues

Units used in biochemistry

IU or U	international unit
mmol	millimole
mmol/l	millimole per litre
nmol	nanomole
µmol	micromole

Common abbreviations used in laboratory results

d, deci	10^{-1} (divided by 10)
f, femto	10^{-15} (divided by 1000 000 000 000 000)
g/dl	grams per decilitre
g/l	grams per litre
IU/l	international units per litre
m, milli	10^{-3} (divided by 1000)
mg/ml	milligrams per millilitre
mm³	cubic millimetre
mU/l	milliunits per litre
n, nano	10^{-9} (divided by 1000 000 000)
p, pico	10^{-12} (divided by 1000 000 000 000)
µ, micro	10^{-6} (divided by 1000 000)

TERMINOLOGY

Abscess	collection of pus in a cavity.
Acid-fast bacteria	takes up the acid stain.
Aerobic bacteria	type of bacteria which requires O_2 to maintain its life.
Airborne or droplet infection	transmission of infection via the air as tiny droplets.
Anaerobic bacteria	type of bacteria that thrives in the absence of O..
Animal vectors	infection transmitted from animals, e.g. rabies from cats, foxes etc.
Campylobacter	type of bacteria which causes food poisoning.
Carbuncle	a boil discharging through many open-
Communicable	transmissible from one person to another by either direct or indirect contact.
Contact	direct or indirect (see Contagious and Fomites).
Contagious	transmitted by direct contact with a person or fomites.
Coombs' test	test for Rhesus incompatibility.
Diplococcus	bacteria which are like berries and are found in pairs.
Endemic	a disease always present in an area.
Epidemic	a disease attacking a large number of people at one time in an area.
Escherichia coli	type of bacillus bacteria responsible for some-types of food poisoning, normally found in the bowel; can cause illness when present elsewhere in the body. Type E0157:H7 is responsible for virulent illness.
Exudation	oozing of fluid into, and out of, capillaries.
Fibrosis	excessive formation of fibrous tissue.
Fomites	objects which are contaminated with organisms of disease, e.g. a toy from a child with chicken-pox.
Fulminating	sudden onset of an infection which is rapid in its course.
Gangrene	death of a piece of body tissue.
Gram-negative bacteria	do not take up Gram stain.
Gram-positive bacteria	take the Gram stain into their cell.
Granulation	healing of a wound where capillaries and other tissues renew from the surface.
Haemolytic	type of bacteria

Haemolytic streptococcus	type of bacteria which causes sore throats and wound infections.
Healing by first intention	edges of clean wound heal together side by side - little scarring.
by second intention	edges of a wound not held together; gap between forms granular tissue before upper skin can grow across the wound.
Herpes zoster	shingles.
Immunoglobulins	antibodies of various types, i.e. IgM, IgG, IgA, IgD and IgE.
Infection	the successful invasion, establishment and growth of micro-organisms in the body.
Infectious	disease transmissible from one host to another.
Infectious parotitis	mumps.
Infestation	the presence of animal parasites in, or on, a living body.
Inflammation	reaction of living tissues to injury, infection or irritation (a body defence).
Insect vectors	transmission of infection via insects, e.g. flies, lice.
Keloid scar	overgrowth of scar tissue forming an elevated ridge.
Koplik's spots	small white spots found on the mucous membranes of the mouth – indicative of measles (morbilli).
Legionella	organism which causes legionnaire's disease.
Lymphadenitis	inflamed lymph gland.
Lymphangitis	inflammation of lymph vessel as infection spreads.
Morbilli	measles.
Necrosis	death of tissue.
Pandemic	as epidemic, but worldwide.
Parotitis (infectious)	mumps.

Paul-Bunnell test	serology test for glandular fever.
Pertussis	whooping cough.
Phagocytosis	the action of the white blood cells which engulf foreign particles of bacteria etc.
Pus	yellowish liquid composed of bacteria and dead leucocytes - the result of infection.
Putrefaction	breaking down of tissue by bacteria accompanied by offensive odour, due to gases produced.
Pyaemia	pus in the blood stream.
Resolution	subsidence of an infection (recovery).
Rose-Waaler or Waaler-Rose test	blood test for rheumatoid arthritis.
Rubella	German measles.
Salmonella	type of bacillus bacteria which causes food poisoning, including typhoid fever.
Septicaemia	bacteria multiply in the blood stream.
Slough	dead tissue which separates from healthy tissue in a wound.
Sporadic	disease occurring in isolated cases.
Staphylococcus	bacteria which are shaped like berries and are found in clusters.
Staphylococcus aureus	type of bacteria which causes food poisoning, skin and wound infections and sore throats.
Streptococcus	bacteria which are shaped like berries and are found in chains.
Suppuration	formation of pus.
Toxaemia	generalised spread of toxins (poisons) in the body - products from bacteria or other invasive micro-organisms.
Varicella	chicken-pox.
Viraemia	viruses circulating and multiplying in the blood stream.

Waterborne or faecal infection	transmission of infection via contaminated water usually taken in by eating or drinking.
WR and Kahn tests	blood tests for syphilis.

Classification of bacteria

-bacillus	bacteria which are rod-shaped.
-coccus	types of bacteria which are round-shaped (like berries).

Spirochaete	shaped like a corkscrew.
Vibrio	bacterium shaped like a comma.

Bacteria are also classified by the stains which they absorb and which show under the microscope, e.g.

Acid fast bacillus	takes up the acid stain
Gram-negative (-ve) **bacteria**	does not take the gram stain
Gram-positive bacteria (+ve)	takes the gram stain

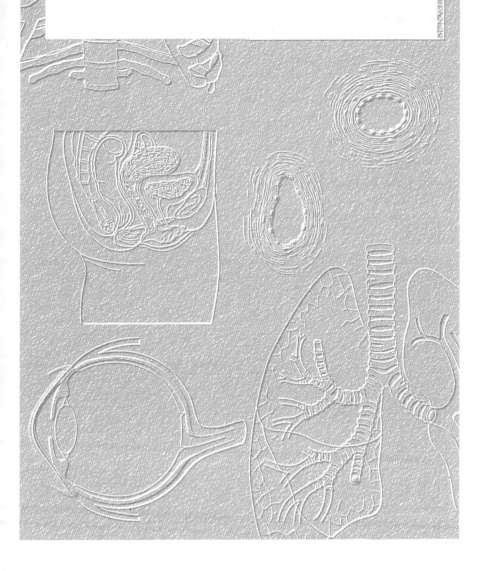

A drug is any substance which, when taken into the body or onto its surface, alters the body's structure or function.

Drugs or medicines are powerful chemicals and the greatest care must be taken to avoid **abuse** or **misuse** of these substances. Dependency or addiction may be physical or psychological. Prevention of abuse is an important responsibility of the doctor and his/her staff.

Misuse or abuse of drugs within medicine refers to any drug that is used in any other way than that for which it is intended.

LEGAL RESPONSIBILITY

Drugs used in medicine are subject to legislation, introduced to prevent harmful or illegal use of these substances. Various regulations have been drawn up and **must** be followed. The doctor is legally responsible for that which he prescribes, and also for the storage and disposal of any drugs within his control. The main legislation involved is:

- The *Medicines Act* 1968
- The *Misuse of Drugs Act* 1971 and its subsequent MODA regulations.

The *Medicines Act* 1968

This includes **all** drugs used in medicine and is concerned with their manufacture, supply, use and storage. It divides medicines into three categories:

1. **General Sales List (GSL)** - those which can be sold over the counter at retail stores, no pharmacist needed. Small quantities only and must be in childproof containers (foil packs accepted), e.g. up to 16 aspirin or paracetamol. There is a list of drugs.

2. **Pharmacy Only Drugs (P)** - all other medicinal products which are not on the GSL and are marked with a P. **Pharmacist must be present for sale** (on premises). Includes small quantities (up to 32 tablets of aspirin and paracetamol), some antihistamines etc.

3. **Prescription Only Medicines (POM)** - lists products which may only be supplied with a prescription. Includes antidepressants, antibiotics, ampoules etc. Large quantities of paracetamol and aspirin are now included in this category. **Controlled drugs** are also included, but these have added requirements under MODA. Marked with POM.

The Misuse of Drugs Act (MODA) 1971 (and subsequent regulations)

This Act controls the manufacture, supply, storage and prescribing of so-called **controlled drugs**, i.e. drugs of addiction. They are classified into various schedules according to their potential for addiction. There are five schedules, the most important in medicine being schedules two and three.

Schedule one (S1) is concerned with drugs not used in medicine, e.g. LSD, marijuana etc. **It is an offence to possess them without a special licence from the Home Office**.

Schedule two (S2) includes derivatives of opium, such as morphine and heroin (diamorphine), as well as cocaine and amphetamines.

Schedule three (S3) includes most barbiturates, minor stimulants, and the tranquilliser Temazepam.

Drugs in schedules two and three are known as **controlled drugs**.

Stringent rules must be observed for these prescriptions and for storage of the drugs within Schedules two and some in three. **No 'repeat' prescribing of these drugs is allowed.**

Schedule four (S4) includes anabolic steroids and tranquillisers, e.g. diazepam. There are no special prescribing requirements at present for these drugs.

Schedule five (S5) contains drugs which have a very small amount of schedule two or three in their formula, e.g. codeine compound tablets. There are no special requirements at present for these drugs within these regulations, although a pharmacist must be present for their sale.

Controlled drugs

Controlled drugs also have very strict requirements concerning both supply and disposal. A special **register** is required for supply of schedule 2 drugs. Invoices for controlled drugs (S2 & S3) and S5 should be kept for 2 years. It is unwise for staff to accept any return of controlled drugs from a patient and they should be referred to the dispensing pharmacist or GP.

Prescriptions for controlled drugs

Controlled drugs for schedule 2 and schedule 3 (see The *Misuse of Drugs Act* 1971, Section 18) have very stringent requirements for prescriptions. These must be prepared by the doctor who is prescribing.

The following requirements are in addition to those for ordinary prescriptions (see later):

- It must be written throughout in the **doctor's own handwriting**.
- **Name and address** of patient.
- The **form and strength** of preparation.
- **Total quantity** of preparation or number of dose units in words and figures.
- The date on the script must be the **date that the prescription is signed**.

The prescribing doctor must be known to the dispensing pharmacist so that his writing and signature are recognised. **It is an offence for a doctor to issue an incomplete prescription for these drugs and the pharmacist must not dispense it.** No repeats are allowed on the same prescription.

There are other rules concerning **instalments** of the drug being issued, and the issuing of quantities to travellers going abroad is limited to 15 days' supply.

A prescription for a controlled drug is valid for 13 weeks, whereas for an ordinary prescription it is for six months.

Phenobarbitone

*Although barbiturates are controlled drugs, phenobarbitone is **exempt** from the strict rules of handwriting by the doctor. It **can** be placed on a computer and printed, **but** the date must be handwritten at the time of signing. This drug is extensively used to control epilepsy.*

N.B. Any prescription for a controlled drug should be placed in a sealed envelope and locked in a drawer or other safe place while awaiting collection.

Temazepam is exempt from **all** special writing requirements for prescription **but** special storage requirements are applicable.

Rules for prescriptions

The following details must be included on all prescription forms (FP10) which must be written in ink or be otherwise indelible:

- Full **name and address** of patient.
- **Age** of patient if under 12 years (legal requirement).
- **Name of drug**.
- **Form of drug**.
- **Strength of drug**.
- **Dosage of drug** with instructions to patient on administration.
- **Quantity of drug** to be dispensed or number of days' treatment in box provided.
- **Signature** in ink by the prescriber.
- **Date** of signing.

The directions to the patient **should never** say simply 'as directed' as this can lead to mistakes being made.

The name, address and telephone number of the doctor prescribing, together with his HA number, will be printed or stamped on the prescriptions supplied by the HA. **Private prescriptions**, often written on the doctor's headed notepaper, **must always** contain the doctor's name, qualifications, address and telephone number.

Supply of NHS prescription pads FP10

These are supplied to GPs directly by the HA. Each prescription is already **printed** with the name, address and telephone number of the doctor. Also included is the doctor's HA number. All now carry a serial number.

Repeat prescriptions

Patients on long-term medication form a large part of the GP's prescribing requirement (see Figure 53). It is essential that certain rules are

FP10 NC

Do you (the patient) have to pay for this prescription?

NO [X] fill in **Parts 1** *and* **3**   YES [X] fill in **Parts 2** *and* **3**
    Give all details we ask for   See notes at bottom of page

Part 1 — For patients who do not have to pay

The patient does not have to pay because he/she

A	[X]	is under 16 years of age
B	[X]	is 16, 17 or 18 *and* in full-time education
C	[X]	is 60 years of age or over
D	[X]	has a maternity exemption certificate
E	[X]	has a medical exemption certificate
F	[X]	has a prescription prepayment certificate
G	[X]	has a War/MoD exemption certificate No:
H	[X]	*gets Income Support *Give details of person getting benefit. This may be your partner. Checks may be made with the DSS.
I	[X]	*gets Family Credit Name:
J	[X]	*gets Disability Working Allowance Date of birth: / /
K	[X]	*gets Income-based Jobseeker's Allowance
L	[X]	*has a current HC2 charges certificate
X	[X]	was prescribed a free-of-charge contraceptive

Now fill in Part 3

Part 2 — For patients who have to pay

I have paid £ _____ for this prescription

Now fill in Part 3

Part 3 — Your declaration

I am the [X] patient [X] patient's representative
I declare that the information is true and complete

Name *In capitals* _____

Address *If different from overleaf* _____

Postcode _____

Signed _____   Date / /

WARNING : FALSE INFORMATION MAY LEAD TO PROSECUTION

- Leaflet HC11 tells you if you are entitled to free prescriptions. It is available from most pharmacies and all main Post Offices. Medical conditions that entitle you to free prescriptions are listed in HC11.
- If you think you may be entitled to free prescriptions, pay *now* and get an NHS receipt (FP57). It tells you how to get your money back.

NAME

Age if under 12 years
yrs. mths. Address

Pharmacy Stamp

Pharmacist's pack & quantity endorsement | No. of days treatment N.B. Ensure dose is stated | NP | Pricing Office use only

Signature of Doctor | Date

For phar-macist No. of Prescns. on form

IMPORTANT:- Read the notes overleaf before going to the pharmacy   Form FP10 NC (Rev. 98)

Figure 53 - Example of a prescription form FP10 NC.

followed to prevent dependency occurring and also to monitor compliance by the patient, i.e. taking the required amount of medication at the correct intervals.

Regular review of prescribing and examination of the patient by the doctor will also highlight any side-effects produced by the treatment being given. Requests to see the patient before the next prescription is supplied may be placed on the computerised slip accompanying the prescription.

PROCEDURES FOR REPEAT PRESCRIPTIONS

In many general practices the receptionist will be involved in the process of the provision of 'repeat prescriptions'. Prescriptions must **never** be signed by the doctor before all details have been entered.

It is essential that a recognised procedure for repeat prescriptions is adopted by every GP and that the staff involved are aware of the part they must play in its implementation.

The procedures for repeat prescriptions may be divided into the following stages:

- requests,
- preparation,
- storage and collection.

REQUESTS

Minimum period of notice

Most surgeries require a minimum period of notice for these prescriptions but it must always be flexible. There are always circumstances where it is imperative that a patient does not miss dosages of their prescribed drugs, e.g. conditions of epilepsy, asthma etc.

Methods of request

These may be by the provision of a computerised 'tear-off' sheet from the presciption or special card provided to the patient by the doctor, listing all repeat medications to be provided. The patient may bring it in person or post it, stating which drugs are required. A stamped addressed envelope may also be provided for return of the new prescription.

Alternatively, patients may telephone a request. This should then be written in a special book or in the general message book according to the practice policy. Writing messages on scraps of paper should be avoided. If telephones are involved, a special number should be used especially for this purpose. This should never be listed in the telephone book, as addicts can easily use this method to try to obtain illegal supplies.

Telephone requests are prone to errors and for this reason many GPs do not encourage this method. Although nowadays most prescriptions are computer-generated, handwritten ones are required if the computer fails, or in emergencies.

PREPARATION

Methods of preparing repeat prescriptions (manual) on FP10 NC green

The following procedures should be followed:

- Check the **notes are correct** for the patient requesting repeat prescription.

- Check that the drug requested **is to be repeated** by checking the patient's request card and notes for the 'rep' instruction.

- Check the **date of the last prescription** and the **amount of drug** given. **Any discrepancy must be reported to the doctor before any script is written.**

- Check if the **review date is due**. If so a note must be attached to the prescription requesting the patient to make an appointment to see the doctor **before** requesting the next prescription.

- Write the prescription following the entry on the **notes and request card** - ensure spelling of drug, dosages and total quantity are all correct, **nothing that**

the doctor has written on the card or notes should be altered in any way.

- Ideally, instructions should not be abbreviated, but should be **written in full**, e.g. twice a day. Care should be taken with decimal points, e.g. '.5' should be written as '0.5' but only when the dosage cannot be expressed as milligrams or micrograms (e.g.'0.5 g' will become '500 mg').

- The strengths microgram and nanogram, **should never be abbreviated** (death of patients has resulted with errors made because this has been mistaken for milligram). Similarly, the word 'units' must **not** be abbreviated.

- If the doctor does not wish the drug to be named on the label when it is dispensed, the **NP box** must be cancelled by striking it through with a line.

- A maximum of **three items** is recommended to be placed on one prescription form. Any space underneath the written instructions should be cancelled with a **diagonal line or Z pattern** to fill the space. This prevents unauthorised addition at a later date

- The request card and the notes should all have entries made with the **date, drug** and **amount** as a record of prescribing

If there are any queries or discrepancies, the doctor must be informed before any prescription is issued.
The prepared prescription should now be placed, together with the patient's notes, ready for signing by the appropriate doctor.

Preparing computerised repeat prescriptions (on FP10 C green)

The drugs required by individual patients will have already been entered into the particular system used by the practice, usually by the doctor. A procedure for these computerised prescriptions should have been agreed with the doctor, and it should ensure safety and prevention of drug abuse similar to the process for manual repeat prescriptions.

Care must be taken to ensure that it is the correct patient's computer file that is accessed. It is also important that a routine check is made each time a prescription is processed to ensure that the drug is authorised and that it is due by date etc.

The number of items on the script can be entered on the prescription at the bottom of the completed items section, or the space can be cancelled by other printed signs, so preventing unauthorised additions.

Entries should also be made in the patient's notes (or other permanent record) stating dates and quantities of the drug concerned for recording purposes.

The accompanying sheet with the computerised prescription may be used for many purposes and can be given to the patient as a future request slip. However, no code must appear on this sheet. If used for any other purpose it should be marked 'CONFIDENTIAL'.

No alterations must be made to a computerised prescription. If there are any mistakes a new prescription must be printed.

Names of controlled drugs must not be placed on computers or printed in any form (see exceptions of phenobarbitone and Temazepam). The requirements for the doctor's own name, address etc. are the same as with ordinary prescriptions:

Reference books

The main reference books used in prescribing are the *British National Formulary* (now also available for use with computers) and *MIMS* (*Monthly Index of Medical Specialities*) a book of proprietary preparations published on behalf of drug companies.

The *BPC* or *British Pharmaceutical Codex* is the official publication on drugs. *The ABPI Compendium of Data Sheets and Summaries of Product Characteristics*, supplied by the pharmaceutical companies in the UK, contains information on storage, legal requirements, drug categories and overdose etc. *The Drug Tariff* from the Prescription Pricing Authority for the Department of Health, contains information on the 'blacklist', i.e. drugs not available on the NHS, 'endorsement' requirements, prescribable appliances and prescription charges, and is updated each month and supplied free to GPs.

Food substances - borderline substances

Prescriptions for these substances, which are foods and not drugs, e.g. soya milk, must have 'ACBS' (Advisory Committee on Borderline Substances) marked on the prescription or they will not be dispensed.

Dressings and appliances

Prescriptions for these must be precise and include substances such as **oxygen cylinders**, **surgical hosiery** and **urine testing equipment**. They must always be written on a separate FP10 from drugs.

SLS prescribing for specific conditions

There is a list of specific conditions for which individual patients may receive NHS prescriptions (further information is found in the Drug Tariff list). These prescriptions must be endorsed with SLS (i.e. selected list scheme).

Generic names

This is the official name for the drug, e.g. salbutamol, and the one that doctors are requested to use in prescribing. Many manufacturers produce the substance and so costs are lower. However, the base of the preparation may not be the same as the proprietary brand and it may have different effects on some individuals.

Proprietary names

This is the individual brand or 'trade name' of the drug, e.g. Ventolin, and is usually more expensive than the generic name drugs. However, in a proprietary drug, a standard preparation will be produced to acceptable standards, with which the prescribing doctor will be familiar.

New EEC directives on information

Bubble packs in containers with written information and warnings are being introduced for all tablets and capsules. This will ensure compliance with the new EEC directive which requires information to be provided for the person being dispensed or purchasing medicines. Pharmacists will be able to provide the bubble pack quantity nearest to the amount stated on the prescription. In order to ensure accuracy, care will have to be taken to adjust the patient's repeat prescription records.

Limited list

Since 1985, regulations have been introduced which name a list of preparations which are **not** allowed to be prescribed on the NHS as they were considered too expensive and many had cheaper generic equivalents. It is known as the limited list and also as the **blacklist**. This includes preparations such as proprietary pain-killers (analgesics), e.g. Disprin, as well as other types of drugs. Should these be accidentally pre-scribed, the doctor will be charged for the prepa-ration him/herself.

PACT (prescribing analysis and cost) and PPA

Information is issued to each general practice at regular intervals from the Prescription Pricing Authority (PPA), comparing the prescribing habits of the doctor with the average for the area.

Practice formulary

Many practices will have a practice formulary. This is a standard list of drugs in different categories, produced by the practice. The list will be the first choice of drugs to be prescribed by the doctors for various conditions from which patients may be suf-fering. Partners will all have agreed to the choice of drugs within it. All practices will have a practice formulary as part of their budgeting process.

STORAGE AND COLLECTION OF REPEAT PRESCRIPTIONS

The following rules apply:

- The signed prescriptions should be placed in an appropriate box away from the reach of anyone coming to the reception desk. They must **never** be left for patients to help themselves.
- The identity of the person collecting the prescription must be **verified**, e.g. request for a date of birth or a middle name etc. of the patient for whom it is written.
- Ensure two pages are **not** stuck together.
- Take care that it is the correct prescription for the **correct** patient - verify address, spelling etc.
- Repeat prescriptions should **not** be hand-ed to children unless the doctor or parent has made special provision.
- All uncollected prescriptions should be **locked away at night** and when the desk is unattended.

Prescriptions directed to outside pharmacies

Some general practices have arrangements with local pharmacists for prescriptions to be sent directly to the pharmacist ready for dispensing. If this procedure is in force it is **essential** that indi-vidual patients have signed that they consent to this arrangement.

Exemptions from prescription charges

Certain categories of patients are exempt from prescription charges, these include those aged under-16 and the over-60s, pregnant women and those patients suffering from some named chron-ic conditions:

- **Colostomy**, **tracheostomy** or **ileostomy** patients.
- **Epilepsy**, on continuous anticonvulsant treatment.
- **Diabetes mellitus**, unless the treatment is by diet alone.
- Patients requiring supplemental **thyrox-ine**.
- **Hypoparathyroidism**.
- **Diabetes insipidus** or **hypopituitarism**.
- **Hypoadrenalism** including **Addison's disease**.
- **Myasthenia gravis**.

The details of other exemptions are to be found on the back of an FP10 form. Many patients may require assistance from the receptionist with the completion of this form.

MEASURES TAKEN TO RECOGNISE DRUG ADDICTS

GPs have a legal obligation to report the name of anyone whom they suspect of being a drug addict. This must be reported to the Medical Officer at the Home Office within seven days. Special FP10 (MDA) prescription forms are used by GPs for prescribing controlled drugs to addicts in instalments. There are 10 light blue double-sided, numbered forms in each pad.

Letters are sent from each HA, warning GPs of suspicious people in the area. This is in order that the doctor may be aware of a partic-ular ruse used to obtain drugs by that person. If the receptionist has any suspicions about some-one visiting the premises, s/he should immedi-ately inform the practice manager or doctor.

The regular review of repeat prescribing for all patients plus the alertness of the receptionist involved in writing repeat prescriptions, helps in the prevention and awareness of any abuse of drugs.

SECURITY OF THE PREMISES

A good burglar alarm system is vital and the surgery window curtains are usually drawn back at night and lights left on so that policemen are able to inspect premises more easily.

FURTHER REQUIREMENTS TO PREVENT DRUG ABUSE

FP10 prescription pads are now designed to prevent unauthorised alteration and photocopying. Special print and coloured paper are used for various categories of prescription. Special inscriptions, visible only in UV light, also aid detection of forgeries. All prescriptions now include serial numbers.

Batches of prescription pads, delivered to the surgery from the HA, should be checked to ensure that all are present. Any discrepancy must be reported to the HA and the police. All unused prescription pads must be stored in a safe place and should be locked away at night and when the doctor's room is unattended. Should any prescriptions be stolen there is a procedure for writing all future prescriptions in red. This is for a stated period of time. It alerts the pharmacist to the possibility of an illegal script.

Drugs should not be stored in cupboards where patients have access, e.g. in the waiting room. Clear directions must be given to patients concerning the dosage and mode of administration. Drug storage cupboards should be locked and should not be marked. The controlled drugs (CD) cupboard keys should be kept on the person of a suitable member of staff, usually the doctor and the practice nurse.

If the doctor's bag contains drugs (as is usual) it must be kept locked and in a safe place. If controlled drugs are contained in the bag, a locked car is not recognised as being a sufficiently secure place. **It must be locked in the case in the locked boot of the car.** Prescription pads should **never** be left in a car where the public may see them.

Any drugs left in the doctor's room, e.g. by drug firm representatives, should be collected and locked away in the appropriate place (usually by the practice nurse).

DISPOSAL OF DRUGS

Drugs are sometimes returned to the surgery by patients. These should be returned to the pharmacist or placed in the special collection service provided by some HAs. This complies with the requirements of the Environmental Protection Act. Controlled drugs have stringent requirements and should only be handled by appropriate designated staff. Returned drugs must never be reused. Expired drugs should be disposed of in the same way. **These drugs must never be mixed with other batches of drugs already in the surgery, for re-use.**

FURTHER INFORMATION

CSM reporting of adverse reactions

Reporting on the 'yellow form' to the CSM (Committee on the Safety of Medicines) via the MCA (**Medical Control Agency**) is an important part of research in general practice and can help to avoid another thalidomide disaster, i.e. the deformities produced in children born to mothers who had been prescribed this drug during pregnancy in the late 1950s and early 60s.

New drugs are always monitored in this way and are marked with a black triangle for the first 2 years following the release to the public on prescription, in order to alert the doctor to the necessity of reporting *any* untoward side-effects.

Nurse practitioners and community nurses

Some of these personnel have been given the legal right to prescribe certain drugs directly to patients. The nurse's UKCC PIN number must be included on the prescription as well as the practice identification number and address.

Practice nurses qualified as District Nurses or Health Visitors who have attended an approved nurse prescribers' course may prescribe from a limited list of drugs (see BNF or Drug Tariff). The FP10 PN used is coloured lilac. Community Nurses and Health Visitors who have also attended the required course may prescribe from same list on FP10 CN which is coloured grey.

Private prescriptions

These may be required when substances are not available on the NHS. All requirements for prescriptions are as for the Medicines Act. Private headed notepaper is normally used and the name and qualifications are required, as well as all other details as already stated for other medicines. Charges are suggested in the BMA list.

ABBREVIATIONS

HRT	hormone replacement therapy
NHS	not available on the NHS

NIDDM	non-insulin dependent diabetes mellitus
IDDM	insulin dependent dia-betes mellitus
NSAID	nonsteroidal anti-inflam-matory drug
OP	original pack (manufac-turer's own pack)
SSRI	selective serotonin reup-take inhibitor (antide-pressant)
TTA	to take away
▲	special reporting requirements

Prescriptions

Abbreviation	Latin	Meaning
a.a.	ana	of each - equal amount
a.c.	ante cibum	before food
alt die	alt die	alternate days
alt noct.	alt nocte	alternate nights
b.d.	bis die	twice daily
c.	cum	with
ex. aq.	ex aquain	water
h.n.	hac nocte	tonight
mane	mane	in the morning
nocte	nocte	at night
NP	nomen proprium	proper name
o.m.	omni mane	every morning
o.n.	omni nocte	every night
p.a	parti affectae	to the affected part
p.c.	post cibum	after food
p.r.n.	pro re nata	whenever necessary
q.d.s.	quater die sumendum	four times daily
q.i.d.	quater in die	four times daily
℞	recipe	take
rep.	repetitur	let it be repeated
s.o.s.	si opus sit	if necessary (one dose only)
stat.	statim	at once
t.d.s.	ter die sumendum	three times daily
t.i.d.	ter in die	three times daily

Preparations

caps.		capsules
neb.		nebulizer
occ. or oc.	occulentae	for the eyes

p.o.c.		for the eyes
p.r.	per rectum	via the rectum
p.v.	per vaginam	via the vagina
pessary		for the vagina
suppos.		suppository
tabs.		tablets
tinct.	tincture	tincture
troch.	trochisci	lozenge
ung.	unguentum	ointment
vap.	vapore	vapour

Measurements

g	gram
mg	milligram
ml	millilitre
ng°	nanogram (°**must not be used on prescriptions**)
S.I.	International System
μg°	microgram (°**must not be used on prescriptions**)

TERMINOLOGY

Classification of drugs etc.

Continuous subcutaneous infusion	drugs given into the layer under the dermis via a syringe driver or 'pump'.
Intradermal (ID)	into the skin.
Intramuscular (IM)	into the muscle.
Intravenous (IV)	via the vein.
Materia medica	drugs used in medicine.
Oral	by mouth.
Parenteral	drugs administered, other than by the oral route.
Pharmacologist	specialist in drugs.
Pharmacology	study of drugs.
Systemic	by injection - affects whole body.

Types of preparation

Elixir	a sweetened aromatic sub-stance containing alcohol.
Enema	a liquid substance inserted into the rectum.
Lavage	a washout - fluid insert-ed through a tube usual-ly into the stomach to remove contents.
Linctus	sweet syrupy liquid for coughs.
Pessary	solid form of drug insert-ed in the vagina (PV).

Suppository	solid form of drug insert-ed in the rectum (PR).	**Chemotherapy**	toxic drugs which are given to kill malignant cells.
Tincture	solution of a drug in alcohol.	**Contraceptive**	drug which prevents conception.

Drug types (classification)

ACE inhibitor	drug which is used for treatment of hyperten-sion or heart failure.	**Cytotoxic**	drugs which kill cells - used to treat malignant disease by killing cancer-ous cells.
Anaesthetic	drug for removal of feel-ing.	**Decongestant**	drug which relieves con-gestion of mucous mem-branes.
General	to the whole body - pro-duces unconsciousness.	**Depressant**	a drug which depresses function of the central nervous system.
Local	to a part - produces numbness.	**Diuretic**	drug which increases the production of urine.
Analgesic	drug for relief of pain.		
Antacid	a substance which neu-tralises stomach acid.	**Expectorant**	liquid form of drug which encourages cough-ing up of secretions from the respiratory tract.
Anti-arrhythmic	drug which controls abnor-mal rhythm of the heart.		
Antibiotic	drug which kills bacteria.	**Hypnotic**	drug which induces sleep.
Anticoagulant	drug which reduces clot-ting.	**Miotic**	for the eyes - to constrict the pupil.
Antidepressant	drug which lifts the patient's mood.	**Mydriatic**	for the eyes - to dilate the pupil.
Anti-emetic	drug which reduces nau-sea.	**Narcotic**	drug derived from opium which will induce deep sleep.
Antihistamine	drug which reduces pro-duction of histamine - for allergies.	**Prophylactic**	a substance used to pre-vent disease.
Antihypertensive	drug which reduces blood pressure.	**Proton pump inhibitor**	drugs which inhibit the production of hydrochlo-ric acid in the stomach.
Anti-inflammatory	drug which reduces inflammation.		
Anti-obesity	drug which helps reduce weight.	**Sedative**	a drug which lowers function.
Antipyretic	drug which reduces fever.	**Steroids**	drugs containing hor-mones - usually of the adrenal cortex.
Antispasmodic	drug which reduces spasms of muscle, e.g. colic.	*Corticosteroids*	drugs from the cortex of the adrenal glands or syn-thetic preparations, which reduce inflammation etc., e.g. prednisolone.
Antitussic	drug which reduces coughing.		
Anxiolytic	drug which reduces anxi-ety.	**Stimulant**	a drug which increases function of the central nervous system.
Beta-blocker	drug which lowers blood pressure etc. - by affect-ing specific beta-nerve receptors.	**Tranquilliser**	a drug which reduces anxiety.
Bronchodilator	drug which dilates the bronchial tubes as in treatment for asthma.	**Vaccine**	a substance prepared specially to stimulate the body to produce its own antibodies or antitoxins.
Carminative	drug which reduces flat-ulence (wind).		

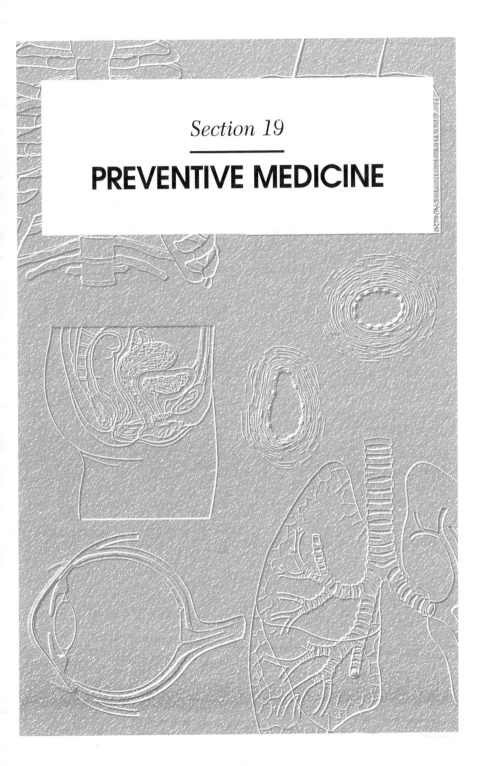

Section 19

PREVENTIVE MEDICINE

HEALTH

The World Health Organisation's definition of health states:

> 'Health is a state of complete physical, mental and social well-being and not merely the absence of disease or infirmity. . . Good Health is held to be fundamental to all peace and security.'

This is the ideal state and is very difficult to achieve.

Each one of the three factors (physical, mental, or social) will affect the other two, e.g. problems with physical health will cause mental and social problems for the patient; similarly, problems with social factors will affect mental and physical well-being.

Preventive medicine is concerned with the prevention of disease in all forms. It is aimed at all people worldwide of all age ranges, not just the 'third world' countries. Based on the concept of 'prevention is better than cure', it is intended to provide a better span and quality of life for human beings wherever possible. It is also considered cheaper to prevent disease than cure it. Prevention can be divided into three main categories:

1. **Primary prevention**
2. **Secondary prevention**
3. **Tertiary prevention**

Primary prevention

This is the complete **avoidance** of the disease, e.g. by immunisation and lifestyle modifications.

Secondary prevention

This is concerned with the **early detection** of disease in patients who have no symptoms, e.g. screening of babies, cervical cytology etc. All screening processes are secondary prevention.

Tertiary prevention

This is concerned with the **limitation of chronic disease** by the discovery and management of the disease before complications have produced disability or handicap, for instance careful management of diabetes mellitus, hypertension and asthma.

DATA

The setting up of **age-sex registers** and use of Read codes on computers are essential tools for the implementation of preventive medicine in general practice.

Read codes provide a clinical coding system on the data of patients, concerning disease, drugs, etc. These systems enable easy recall of information which can be used for research, statistics and regular recall of patients.

PRIMARY HEALTH-CARE TEAM (PHCT)

The primary health-care team (PHCT) is a group of professional health-care workers within the community, each contributing their own special skills to the benefit of patients' well-being. They are normally the first professionals involved in the care of the patient.

In general practice, it is the PHCT who is at the front line of preventive medicine. This aspect has been given a definite emphasis since the 1990 GP Contract. More requirements, including introduction of immunisation targets and the screening of elderly people, are now included in the Terms and Conditions of Service for GPs.

Goals

It is important that the PHCT work together as a team towards a common goal. Each member should be aware of the specialist skills provided by each of the other members, thus providing support to each other and the best care for the patient. It is always important to remember what the overall achievement should be, i.e. **the best care of the patient**.

Among the common goals is that of preventive medicine. The new 'primary-care groups' (PCGs) include all disciplines and should help to achieve the aims of the 1998 Green Paper 'Our Healthier Nation'.

Members

The basic PHCT is composed of:

- **GP**
- **Health visitor**
- **Community nurse/midwife**
- **Practice nurse**

The administrative support from the **practice manager**, **receptionists** and **secretaries** (who are also members of the team) is absolutely vital and ensures the smooth running of the team. Good communication is vital and it is here that the receptionist can bring invaluable support by ensuring accuracy in conveying messages.

The other specialist members of the primary team include:

- **Counsellors**
- **Social workers**
- **Community psychiatric nurses**
- **School nurses**
- **Continence advisors**
- **Chiropodists**
- **Dietitians**
- **Domiciliary physiotherapists**
- **Occupational therapists**
- **Speech therapists**
- **Orthoptists**
- **Pharmacists**
- **Dental officers**

AREAS OF PRIMARY PREVENTIVE MEDICINE

These include:

- **Immunisation**
- **Public health and housing controls**
- **Health education**
- **Dental fluoridation**

Immunisation

This is one of the main areas of prevention (see Section 22). Before the advent of immunisation of children against infectious diseases such as diphtheria, many children died before reaching puberty.

Public health and housing controls

Without the sweeping changes in these areas, which came about in the late 19th century ensuring better housing, clean water supplies and disposal of sewage, the general standard of health would be very poor. This should never be underestimated and control of the environment is paramount in the battle for health. Increasing pollution of the atmosphere is producing health hazards for many of the population at the present time.

Health education

This is aimed at persuading people to live healthy lifestyles and take a positive view towards responsibility for their own, and their children's, health. The greatest problem is the 'it won't happen to me' attitude. Anti-smoking, anti-drugs and AIDS campaigns, together with all the other areas in which the Health Education Authority (HEA) is involved, play a major part in these fields. The provision of the many leaflets is of great help to the surgery and to the health visitor in their relationship with the patient.

Health education begins with preconceptual advice and continues through to, and includes, old age. Parents and teachers play a major role in childhood. 'Example' is the greatest teacher of all.

IMPORTANT AREAS OF PREVENTIVE MEDICINE

The following shows areas of health promotion in different sectors of the community:

Maternal care (antenatal and postnatal)

Screening for defects in the fetus and diseases in the mother; early detection or prevention of toxaemia of pregnancy.

Child care

- Detection of abnormalities by **screening tests** - physical, mental and social.
- **Developmental surveillance** - hearing, speech and visual defects etc.
- **Immunisation**.
- Prevention of **accidents** - poisoning etc.
- **Child abuse**, including sexual.
- **Dental caries**.

Adolescents

- **Smoking**.
- **Contraception** and unwanted **pregnancy**.
- **Accidents** at work and home.
- **Alcohol** and **drug abuse**.
- **Sexually transmitted disease** including AIDS.

Adults 16 to 64 years

- Complications of **pregnancy**.
- **Smoking**.
- **Sexually transmitted disease**.
- **Rubella** (German measles).
- **Motor accidents**.
- **Alcohol** and **drug abuse**.
- **Cancer** of the **breast** and **cervix**.
- **Testicular cancer**.
- **Hypertension**.
- **Coronary heart disease**.
- **Suicide**.
- **Cancer of the colon**.

Elderly 65 years and over

- **Hypertension**.
- Loss of **autonomy**.
- **Dementia**.
- **Hearing defects**.
- **Feet problems**.
- **Visual defects**.
- **Influenza**, with emphasis on those at risk due to other diseases.
- **Hypothermia**.
- **Accidents** and **loss of balance**.

The range of preventive medicine is a vast one and these are only examples of the many areas where the individual may benefit from the prevention of cause of disease, health education or screening process.

HEALTH FOR ALL BY THE YEAR 2000

This concerns the challenge by the World Health Organisation (WHO) in 1978 to its member states to achieve '**Health for All by the Year 2000**'. Included are the European countries, and 38 target areas of health are included together with the collective aim of reducing the difference in health status between countries and between groups within the countries. Lower socio-economic classes within countries have been shown to be more susceptible to early death and higher incidence of disease.

Health of the Nation

The UK accepted the challenge and the Government White Paper *Health of the Nation* named specific areas where a concentration of resources for particular preventive measures should actually improve the lifespan and quality of life for the individual.

All needed to play their part in order to achieve the aims within this paper, the government, organisations, agencies, families and the individual.

Named target areas

There were five key areas proposed for initial targeting:

1. **coronary heart disease and stroke**
2. **cancers**
3. **prevention of accidents**
4. **mental illness**

5. HIV/AIDS and sexual health

These targets are based on the criteria of each area being:

- a major cause of premature death, avoidable ill-health and/or disability;
- one where effective intervention was possible;
- one where there was sufficient knowledge of the level of ill-health and scope for making improvements to allow national or local targets to be set and progress towards them monitored.

Targets of *Health of the Nation*

Coronary heart disease and stroke by year 2000

- Cut death rates in under-65s by at least 40%; and 30% for 64- to 74-year-olds.
- Cut death rate for stroke in 65-74s by at least 40%.
- Risk factor target: reduce prevalence of smoking by 35% in men and 29% in women.

Cancers by year 2000

- Breast cancer: cut deaths in 50- to 64-year-olds by 25%.
- Invasive cervical cancer: cut incidence by 20%.

by 2005

- Skin cancer: increase to halt.

by 2010

- Lung cancer: cut deaths in male under 75s by 30% and females by 15%.

Risk-factor targets by 1994

- Cut smoking in 11- to 15-year-olds by at least 33%.

by 2000

- One-third of women smokers to quit smoking at start of pregnancy.
- Cut total cigarette consumption by at least 40%.

Mental illness by 2000

- 'Significantly improve' health and social functioning of mentally ill.
- Suicide: cut overall rate by at least 15% and rate in severely mentally ill by at least 33%.

HIV/AIDS and sexual health

(As it is difficult to quantify the incidence of **HIV** and **AIDS**, a measure is taken against the incidence of another sexually transmitted disease - **gonorrhoea.**)

- By 1995: gonorrhoea - cut incidence in 15- to 64-year-olds by 20%.
- By 2000: conceptions - cut rate in under 16s by at least 50%.
- By 1997: drug misuse - cut numbers sharing needles by at least 50%.
- By 2000: drug misuse - cut by a further 50%.

TARGETS

General practices receive special 'target' payments for health promotion which are associated with *Health of the Nation* requirements. These targets are set locally by discussions between the Health Authority and the doctors' representatives, the Local Medical Committee. The old 'banding system' is no longer applied, and agreed payments are made to practices on an annual basis. Strict **protocols** must be followed by practices and records kept, however the requirement for forms by the Health Authorities has been greatly reduced.

Primary prevention

Target areas include the **reduction of smoking** which will cut related illnesses such as **coronary artery disease** and **lung** and **cervical cancer.**

Secondary prevention

Also targeted are patients who are likely to suffer from **coronary artery disease** and **hypertension.** They are screened and advised before the development of any clinical signs or symptoms of the disease.

Tertiary prevention

Another target area is the minimisation of death and disease through **hypertension, coronary heart disease** (**CHD**) and **strokes.**

Chronic disease management programmes

Practices participate in chronic disease management programmes for **asthma** and **diabetes mellitus.** These are also examples of tertiary preventive medicine.

Asthma

The effective control of asthma will help to prevent unnecessary deaths and give the patient a better quality of life. Early recognition of the need to increase **prophylactic (preventive) treatment** is an essential requirement in this condition.

Diabetes mellitus

Similarly the effective control of this condition will **prevent damage** to many organs, e.g. blood vessels, nervous system, kidneys and eyes.

Priority target groups are identified, i.e. those most at risk in each category. The factors include family history as this is an unavoidable factor in predisposition to disease.

BENEFITS OF STOPPING SMOKING

The benefits of cessation of smoking are:

- A decrease in the ease of blood clotting within two weeks, lowering the risk of **thrombosis**.
- A lowering of **blood cholesterol** to normal for the individual within one month.
- A reduction in the **complications** associated with chronic heart disease within one year.
- A restoration of the **risk of stroke** to 'normal' range within five years; reduction of the chances of **atheroma** (furring up of arteries with fatty deposits).

Passive smoking

The damage suffered through passive smoking is now an accepted fact and parents should be advised on the effect it has on their children.

Lifestyle advice, including smoking, exercise, diet (less fat consumption) and alcohol consumption as well as keeping an 'age/sex' register are included in the requirements for the bandings.

BODY MASS INDEX (BMI) RECORDINGS

The **body mass index** (BMI) of an individual can be used to calculate the obesity risk to health of that individual.

It has long been recognised that there is a correlation between obesity, hypertension and early mortality.

The BMI is calculated with the following formula:

$$\frac{\text{Weight (kilograms)}}{\text{Height (metres) squared}} = \text{BMI}$$

A BMI of 10 to 24.9 is considered acceptable

OPPORTUNISTIC SCREENING

Instead of special health promotion clinics, it is now accepted and recognised that opportunistic screening is more effective in primary and secondary preventive medicine. The GP and his/her staff have always been involved in the routine testing of urine and recording of blood pressure, and cases of diabetes mellitus and hypertension have been regularly detected. Hypertension is a 'silent killer' as no symptoms occur until there has already been extensive damage to the body.

ROLE OF THE RECEPTIONIST IN PREVENTIVE MEDICINE

The receptionist in general practice will be involved in the collection and programming of statistics and also the maintenance of the **age/sex register** or **morbidity register**. Various letters and questionnaires will be required to be given or sent to patients. Efficient recording and filing of notes are essential.

Ensuring there is always a good supply of health education leaflets available for patients, is a valuable contribution to the work of the PHCT. Local health education officers/health promotion agencies will readily supply these on request as well as assist in the setting up of specialist displays on many aspects of preventive medicine.

Immunisation and **cervical smear targets** will also be a priority. An understanding of the reasons for these important requirements will enable the receptionist to assist the PHCT with an even greater motivation.

OUR HEALTHIER NATION

A consultative Green Paper issued by the Government in 1998 entitled 'Our Healthier Nation' stated their intentions for the planned improvement of the nation's health up to the year 2010.

Table 4 – A Contract for Health

Government and National Players can:	Local Players and Communities can:	People can:
Provide national coordination and leadership.	Provide leadership for local health strategies by developing and implementing Health Improvement Programmes.	Take responsibilty for their own health and make healthier choices about their lifestyle.
Ensure that policy making across Government takes full account of health and is well informed by research and the best expertise available.	Work in partnerships to improve the health of local people and tackle the root causes of ill health.	Ensure their own actions do not harm the health of others.
Work with other countries for international cooperation to improve health.	Plan and provide high quality services to everyone who needs them.	Take opportunities to better their lives and their families' lives, through education, training and employment.
Assess risks and communicate those risks clearly to the public.		
Ensure that the public and others have the information they need to improve their health.		
Regulate and legislate where necessary.		
Tackle the root causes of ill health.		

Source: Secretary of State for Health (1998)
Our Healthier Nation: A Contract for Health, 30

Table 5 – Factors affecting health

Fixed	Social and economic	Environment	Lifestyle	Access to services
Genes	Poverty	Air quality	Diet	Education
Sex	Employment	Housing	Physical activity	NHS
Ageing	Social exclusion	Water quality	Smoking	Social services
		Social environment	Alcohol	Transport
			Sexual behaviour	Leisure
			Drugs	

Source: Secretary of State for Health (1998)
Our Healthier Nation: A Contract for Health, 16

The paper states that good health is a top priority for the government. The aim is to prevent people falling ill in the first place by '**tackling the root causes of the avoidable illnesses**' (p.2). In recent years emphasis has been placed on the individual's responsibility to live healthy lives via lifestyle changes. This has been beneficial but has also led to an attitude which blames the individual for his/her poor health. The plan now is for more attention and government action to be placed on **controlling** those factors which damage health and are beyond the individual's control. This is to be a **joint** effort between the government, local communities and individuals in a '**National Contract for Better Health**' (Table 4).

Inequality

Poor health has complex causes, some of which are fixed, such as **genetic factors** and **ageing**. However, many other factors which may cause bad health can be changed, e.g. **lifestyle, diet, physical exercise, sexual behaviour, smoking, alcohol and drugs**. **Social** and **economic** factors also play a part, for instance poverty, unemployment and social exclusion. Our **environment**, including air and water quality, housing, as well as access to good services such as **education**, transport, social services provision and the NHS, all affect our health (Table 5).

Health inequalities are widening:

> '**Poor people are ill more often and die sooner.**' (p.3)

These fundamental inequalities will be concen-

trated on by giving attention and resources to the areas most affected by: air pollution, low wages, unemployment, poor housing, and crime and disorder, all of which can make people both mentally and physically ill.

Linked programmes

A series of programmes linked to improving factors affecting health are to be implemented by the government, including measures on:

- '**Welfare to work**' (Tackling unemployment).
- **Crime**.
- **Housing**.
- **Education**.
- **Health**.

Key aims

There are two key aims for improving the health of the population:

1. '*To improve the health of the population as a whole by increasing the length of people's lives and the number of years people spend free from illness.*'

2. '*To improve the health of the worst off in society and to narrow the health gap.*' (p.14)

The government intends to set out a new way to achieve this goal '**between the old extremes of individual victim blaming**' and '**nanny state social engineering on the other**' (p.5) by introducing the National Contract for Better Health.

Partnerships

The following groups will work together::
- **Government.**
- **Health Authorities.**
- **Local authorities.**
- **Businesses.**
- **Voluntary bodies.**

Government

'The Government will help to assess the risk to health by making sure that people are given information on health which is accurate, understandable and credible. Where there are real threats to health we will not hesitate to take tough action – though regulation and legislation will be the exception, not the rule.' (p.5)

Health Authorities

'Health Authorities will have a key role in leading local alliances to develop Health Improvement Programmes, which will identify local needs and translate the national contract into local action.' (p.5)

Local authorities

'Local Authoities will have a new duty to promote the economic, social and environmental well-being of their areas.' (p.5)

Businesses

'Businesses can bring new skills to bear, including marketing and communications – as well as improving the health and safety of their own employees.' (p.5)

Voluntary bodies

'Voluntary bodies can act as advocates to give powerful voice to local people.' (p.6)

Actions

- Healthy schools, focusing on children (Table 6).
- Healthy workplaces, focusing on adults (Table 7).
- Healthy neighbourhoods, focusing on older people.

Table 6 – Healthy schools

Government can:	Healthy schools can:	Pupils and Parents can:
Set high educational standards. Ensure high quality teaching. Fund safe and healthy school buildings. Establish a National Advisory Group on Personal, Social and Health Education. Establish a healthy schools award scheme.	Give children the capacity to make the most of their lives and their future families' lives. Ensure that children learn about the key influences on their own health. Provide healthy choices and set nutritional standards for school meals. Ensure that pupils take regular exercise and encourage participation in sport. Create an environment that promotes the emotional well-being of the children.	Work together to share responsibilty for academic achievement, healthier eating, better exercises, and a responsible attitude to smoking, drugs, alcohol, sex and relationships. Minimise the use of car journeys to and from school.

Source: Secretary of State for Health (1998) *Our Healthier Nation: A Contract for Health*, 50

Table 7 – Healthy Workplaces

Government can:	Employers can:	Employees can:
Set standards of health and safety in the working environment.	Have excellent standards of health and safety management.	Play their part in following health and safety rules and guidelines.
Ensure minimum employment rights to encourage decent and responsible partnerships between staff and managers.	Take measures to reduce stress at work.	Either directly or through trade union safety representatives, work with employers to create a healthy working environment.
Encourage health at work initiatives through the Health and Safety Executive's *Good Health is Good Business* campaign.	Try to create flexible working arrangements that are compatible with employees' home lives and provide childcare facilities.	Support colleagues who have problems or who are disabled.
Through the Health and Safety Commission, publish a consultation paper on a ten-year strategy for occupational health.	Ensure a smoke-free working environment.	Contribute to charitable and social work through work-based voluntary organisations.
	Contribute to and implement the Health and Safety Commission's forthcoming consultation paper on a ten-year strategy for occupational health.	
	Make healthy choices easy for staff, eg provision for cyclists, healthy canteens.	Source: Secretary of State for Health (1998) *Our Healthier Nation: A Contract for Health*, 51

Targets

Previously set targets will continue. However, based on health statistics of 1996, four priority areas will be targeted for 2010. The new goals are as follows:

1. *Heart disease and stroke*   reduce death rate from heart disease and stroke and related illnesses amongst people aged under 65 years by at least one-third (Table 8).

2. *Accidents*   reduce accidents by at least one-fifth (Table 9).

3. *Cancer*   reduce death rate from cancer amongst people aged under 65 years by at least one-fifth (Table 10).

4. *Mental Health*   reduce death rate from suicide and undetermined injury by at least one-sixth (Table 11).

The government acknowledges that these are tough targets to achieve, but points out that there are strong personal, social and economic arguments for achieving them. At the present time, heart disease, stroke and related illnesses cost the National Health Service an estimated £3.8 billion every year. Approximately 187 million working days are lost every year because of sickness, costing business tax £12 billion. **But above all, the individual and family will experience better health!**

Table 8 – A National Contract on Heart Disease and Stroke

	Government and National Players can:	Local Players and Communities can:	People can:
Social and Economic	Continue to make smoking cost more through taxation. Tackle joblessness, social exclusion, low educational standards and other factors which make it harder to live a healthier life.	Tackle social exclusion in the community which makes it harder to have a healthy lifestyle. Provide incentives to employees to cycle or walk to work, or leave their cars at home.	Take opportunities to better their lives and their families' lives through education, training and employment.
Environmental	Encourage employers and others to provide a smoke-free environment for non-smokers.	Through local employers and others, provide a smoke-free environment for non-smokers. Through employers and staff, work in partnership to reduce stress at work. Provide safe cycling and walking routes.	Protect others from second-hand smoke.
Lifestyle	End advertising and promotion of cigarettes. Enforce prohibition of sale of cigarettes to youngsters. Develop Healthy Living Centres. Ensure access to, and availability of, a wide range of foods for a healthy diet. Provide sound information on the health risks of smoking, poor diet and lack of exercise.	Encourage the development of healthy schools and healthy workplaces. Implement an Integrated Transport Policy, including a national cycling strategy and measures to make walking more of an option. Target information about a healthy life on groups and areas where people are most at risk.	Stop smoking or cut down, watch what they eat and take regular exercise.
Services	Encourage doctors and nurses and other health professionals to give advice on healthier living. Ensure catering and leisure professionals are trained in healthy eating and physical exercise.	Provide help to people who want to stop smoking. Improve access to a variety of affordable food in deprived areas. Provide facilities for physical activity and relaxation and decent transport to help people get to them. Identify those at high risk of heart disease and stroke and provide high quality services.	Learn how to recognise a heart attack and what to do, including resuscitation skills. Have their blood checked regularly. Take medicine as it is prescribed.

Source: Secretary of State for Health (1998) *Our Healthier Nation: A Contract for Health*, 64

Table 9 – National Contract on Accidents

	Government and National Players can:	Local Players and Communities can:	People can:
Social and Economic	Improve areas of deprivation through urban regeneration. Tackle social exclusion and joblessness.	Tackle social exclusion and joblessness in the community.	Take opportunities to combat poverty through education, training and employment.
Environmental	Improve safety of roads. Ensure compliance with seatbelt requirements and other road traffic laws. Help set standards for products and appliances. Promote higher standards of safety management.	Improve facilities for pedestrians and cycle paths. Develop safer routes for schools. Adopt traffic calming and other engineering measures and make roads safer. Work for healthier and safer workplaces. Make playgrounds safe.	Check the safety of appliances and use them correctly. Instal smoke alarms. Drive safely. Take part in safety management in the workplace.
Lifestyle	Provide information on how to avoid osteoporosis so that accidents don't lead to broken bones. Run public safety campaigns. Ensure strategies are coodinated across Government Departments and Agencies. Provide information on ways to avoid accidents.	Ensure those in need have aids to prevent accidents, like car seats for babies. Work for whole school approaches to health and safety. Target accident prevention at those most at risk.	Adopt safe behaviour for themselves and their children. Wear cycle helmets. Wear a seatbelt. Not drink and drive. Keep physically fit. Eat a balanced diet which contains enough calcium and vitamin D, take regular exercise and stop smoking to protect themselves from osteoporosis.
Services	Encourage health professionals to give appropriate advice. Ensure professionals are trained in accident prevention.	Provide appropriate treatment to high-risk groups to prevent osteoporosis.	Have regular eye-tests. Know emergency routine.

Source: Secretary of State for Health (1998) Our Healthier Nation: A Contract for Health, 69

Table 10 – A National Contract on Cancer

	Government and National Players can:	Local Players and Communities can:	People can:
Social and Economic	Continue to make smoking more costly through taxation. Tackle joblessness, social exclusion, low educational standards and other factors which make it harder to live a healthier life.	Tackle social exclusion in the community to make it easier for people to make healthy choices. Work with deprived communities and with businesses to ensure a more varied and affordable choice of food.	Take opportunities to better their lives and their families' lives through education, training and employment.
Environmental	Encourage employers and others to provide a smoke-free environment for non-smokers. Encourage local action to tackle radon in the home. Continue to press for international action to restore the ozone layer.	Through local employers and others, provide a smoke-free environment for non-smokers. Tackle radon in the home.	Protect others from second-hand smoke. Cover up in the sun.
Lifestyle	End advertising and promotion of cigarettes. Prohibit sale of cigarettes to youngsters and ensure enforcement. Support Healthy Living Centres. Provide reliable and objective information on the health risks of smoking, poor diet and too much sun.	Encourage the development of healthy workplaces and healthy schools. Target health information on groups and areas where people are most at risk.	Stop or cut down smoking and watch what they eat. Be careful when they are in the sun and ensure that young children are not exposed to too much sun. Follow sensible drinking advice.
Services	Encourage doctors and nurses and other health professionals to give advice on prevention. Ensure that healthy schools work with pupils and parents to improve health. Implement effective and high-quality cancer screening programmes. Ensure equal access to high-quality treatment and care.	Provide help in stopping smoking to people who want to stop. Improve access and availability to a variety of affordable food in deprived areas. Ensure hard-to-reach groups come forward for cancer screening services. Ensure rapid treatment for cancers when they are diagnosed.	Attend cancer screenings when invited. Seek medical advice promptly if they are wanted.

Source: Secretary of State for Health (1998) *Our Healthier Nation: A Contract for Health*, 75

Table 11 – A National Contract on Mental Health

	Government and National Players can:	Local Players and Communities can:	People can:
Social and Economic	Tackle joblessness, social exclusion and other factors which make it harder to have a healthier lifestyle. Tackle alcohol and drug misuse.	Develop local support networks, eg for recently widowed/bereaved, lone parents, unemployed people and single people. Develop court diversion schemes. Develop job opportunities for people with mental illness. Develop local strategies to support the needs of mentally ill people from black and minority/ethnic groups.	Develop parenting skills. Support friends at times of stress – be a good listener. Participate in support networks. Take opportunities to better their lives and their families' lives through education, training and employment.
Environmental	Continue to invest in housing and reduce homelessness. Encourage employers to address workplace stress. Reduce isolation through transport policy. Promote healthier schools. Address levels of mental illness amongst prisoners.	Develop effective housing strategies. Reduce stress in the workplace. Improve community safety.	Improve workload management.
Lifestyle	Increase public awareness and understanding of mental health. Reduce access to means of suicide. Support Healthy Living Centres.	Focus on particular high-risk groups, eg young men, people in isolated rural communities. Encourage positive local media reporting. Develop and encourage use of range of leisure facilities.	Use opportunities for relaxation and physical exercise and try to avoid using alcohol/smoking to reduce stress. Increase understanding of what good mental health is.
Services	Develop standards and training for primary care and specialist mental health services. Improve recruitment/ retention of mental health professionals. Identify/advise on effective treatment and care. Develop protocols to guide best practice.	Promote high-quality pre-school education and good mental health in schools and promote educational achievement. Ensure mental health professionals are well trained and supported. Develop a range of comprehensive mental health services for all age groups and alcohol and drug services for young people and adults. Support carers of people with long-term disability and chronic illness. Provide advice on financial problems. Develop culturally sensitive services.	Contribute information to service planners and get involved. Contact services quickly when difficulties start. Increase knowledge about self-help. Source: Secretary of State for Health (1998) *Our Healthier Nation: A Contract for Health*, 79

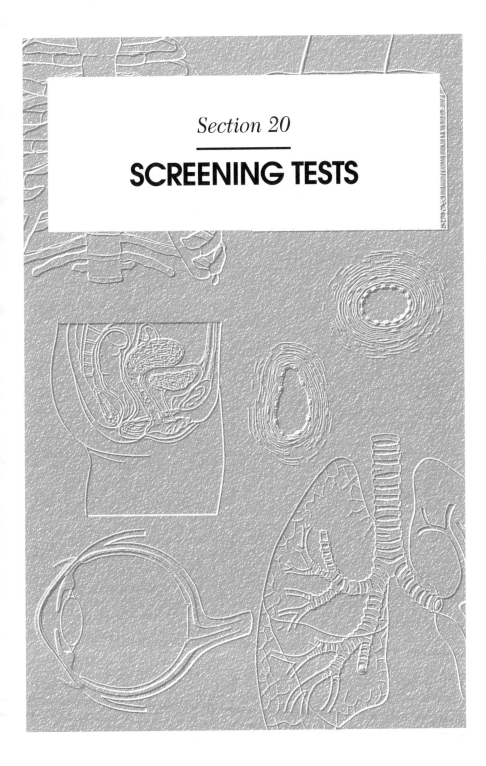

Section 20

SCREENING TESTS

SCREENING

Screening is the detection of disease before the presence of symptoms. It is a form of secondary preventive medicine, aiming to detect the presence or absence of a disease or condition. It may be done on an individual (opportunistic screening at the practice) or through mass screening of the whole population.

The purpose of screening is to prevent early death, reduce disease, and improve the quality of life. The principle is based on the fact that certain diseases and conditions can be recognised by a simple test well before any serious disease has developed or symptoms occurred.

There are certain ethical requirements before screening is approved:

- The disease being searched for should always be a **serious** one.

- The screening test itself should always be **simple** to perform and **not give false results**.

- As far as possible the test should be an **objective rather than a subjective test**; i.e. the results must be clear and not left to individual opinion.

- The test should be **safe** and **not induce undue fear** in people tested; counselling of participants is important, they must understand its nature.

- **Effective treatment** must be available for the disease or condition for which the screening is being performed.

ANTENATAL SCREENING

Tests performed on pregnant women are important in detecting abnormalities of both mother and fetus at an early stage. One of the main aims is to ensure that a healthy baby is born to a healthy mother. The following screening tests are performed:

Urine testing   to detect any abnormal content

e.g. albumin may suggest a urine infection or kidney disease. Its occurrence later in pregnancy may indicate developing toxaemia of pregnancy.

Sugar can indicate diabetes mellitus.

Blood pressure   to detect its state at the start of pregnancy and watch for any sign of hypertension developing - indicative of developing toxaemia of pregnancy (PET see terminology of the female reproductive system, Section 11).

Blood tests

- to determine **blood group** and **Rhesus factor**;

- to detect **anaemia**;

- to detect immunity to **rubella** (German measles);

- to detect **syphilis** if present in order to treat and prevent fetal deformities;

- to detect **hepatitis B** antibodies;

- to detect **HIV** antibodies (not routine but anonymous testing is performed in some areas as a survey);

- to detect **sickle-cell anaemia** and **thalassaemia** (test offered to women of West Indian, African and Mediterranean origin).

An examination per vaginam may be performed at first visit to detect any abnormality of the reproductive system and the size of the uterus.

Later visits

Urine, blood pressure, weight, height of fundus of uterus and any fluid retention (oedema) will be checked at each visit. The main aim of detecting the early onset of **toxaemia of pregnancy** (PET) in order to avoid **eclampsia** where fits occur and death of baby and mother can result, is paramount in antenatal care. Rapid weight gain, fluid retention, albumin in the urine and hypertension are all signs of the developing condition.

Ultrasound scan

Ultrasound waves build up a picture of the fetus in the uterus. This is used to:

- check fetus' **measurements**, size for dates, growth etc.;

- check for **multiple pregnancy**;

- detect **abnormalities**, particularly of head or spine (**spina bifida**);

- check position of placenta (**placenta praevia**).

Procedure

The woman is asked to drink plenty of fluid as a full bladder produces a better picture of the uterus by pushing it up into the abdominal cavity. Jelly is then placed on the abdomen with the patient lying on her back.

An instrument is passed backwards and forwards over the skin and high frequency sound is beamed through the abdomen. This is reflected back and creates a picture on the screen.

Alpha-fetoprotein test

This is a blood test performed at about 16-18 weeks of pregnancy; used to determine the level of alpha-fetoprotein (AFP) in the blood which, if raised, may indicate a **neural-tube defect**, such as **spina bifida** or **ancencephaly** (undeveloped brain). Low levels may suggest other abnormalities such as **Down's syndrome**.

'Triple screening' or 'triple plus' test

This is a blood test for **Down's syndrome**. It combines the levels of AFP with levels of two hormones present in the mother's blood and predicts the likelihood of Down's syndrome.

Amniocentesis

This test may be offered at 12-18 weeks of pregnancy to older women (over 35 years) where the risk of Down's syndrome is higher, or where there is a family history of the condition. Positive testing for spina bifida or Down's syndrome with the AFP test will usually be followed by **amniocentesis**. It produces a very small increase in the risk of abortion.

Procedure

An ultrasound test will first determine the position of the fetus and placenta. After a local anaesthetic, a needle is passed through the wall of the abdomen to withdraw amniotic fluid which surrounds the fetus. This fluid is sent to the laboratory for testing for chemical content and also the genetic content of cells. In Down's syndrome the chromosomes are abnormal - a splitting of number 21 or the presence of an extra chromosome. Other abnormalities will also be investigated.

Chorionic villus sampling

This test, available in some hospitals, can be carried out earlier than amniocentesis at eight to 11 weeks of pregnancy. It has a higher risk of abortion than amniocentesis. It is used to detect:

- **Down's syndrome**,
- inherited diseases, such as **sickle-cell anaemia** or **thalassaemia**,
- some sex-linked diseases, for example **haemophilia**.

It will **not** detect spina bifida. The full effects of this test upon the developing fetus are not yet known.

Procedure

Using ultrasound as a guide, a fine tube is passed through the vagina and cervix, or sometimes through the abdomen, and a small piece of the developing placenta, called **chorionic tissue**, is withdrawn. This is sent to the laboratory for testing.

TESTS ON THE NEWBORN

A baby is completely examined soon after birth, to detect any congenital abnormalities so that measures can be introduced to minimise resulting problems. Conditions such as **club foot** or **cleft palate** are an obvious handicap. The screening for undescended testicles in males and other conditions is continued throughout infancy and childhood.

Apgar rating

This is a test performed on all newborn and involves awarding of a rating for the following:

- **heart rate**
- **respiratory effort**
- **muscle tone**
- **reflex state**
- **colour**

A baby in the perfect state at birth will score two points for each category giving a total score of 10.

This test is repeated at certain intervals following birth. It gives good indication of the probability of developmental problems and/or epilepsy, due to lack of oxygen at birth.

Blood tests

These include blood tests for the detection of:

- Phenylketonuria (**Guthrie test**)
- **Hypothyroidism** or cretinism

The Guthrie test, also known as 'the **heel-prick test**' as the blood is taken from the newborn's heel, is performed after feeding has been established (usually at five days). It is used to detect a chemical known as **phenylketone** which is an abnormality present in babies unable to properly break down certain proteins. If not detected at birth and special diet implemented, it causes damage to mental development.

Hypothyroidism, if detected, can be treated by the administration of thyroxine and the abnormal mental development will be prevented.

The test for **congenital dislocation of hip** is done following birth when the '**click test**' or **Otalani's test** is performed. When the hips are rotated a click is heard if a dislocation is present.

CHILDREN

Screening tests for children are done routinely by the health visitor, medical officer or GP in **child health surveillance**.

These tests are done at different ages, the main concentration being in the infant and preschool periods.

Five main areas are involved for developmental screening:

- **locomotion** and **posture**,
- **muscle control** and **function**,
- **speech** and **language**,
- **growth**,
- **social development**.

Hearing testing is an important area of screening, and **routine testing** is an important tool for preventing loss of language development due to unidentified problems. **Squints** are usually minimised if early detection is made.

ADULT SCREENING

Tests for recognising precancerous conditions are now recommended and include those for **carcinoma of the cervix**, **breast cancer**, **large bowel** and **testicular cancer**.

Screening for coronary heart disease, hypertension and obesity have been discussed in Section 19.

Cervical smears

The '**Pap**' test, named after the man who introduced it - Papanicolaou, is one of the foremost screening tests at present. In England and Wales a programme of screening for women aged from 25 years to 64 years is available on the NHS (20 to 60 years in Scotland), and GP targets for payment are at present set at 80% for the higher level and 50% for the lower. This will exclude those women who have had a hysterectomy with the removal of the cervix. An automatic three-year **recall scheme** is in operation, although some HAs still only recall five-yearly.

The smear must not be taken during menstruation. Cells are removed with a special spatula (Aylesbury) or cytobrush from the area of the cervical canal. It is important that they are removed from the correct area. These are then placed on a glass slide and immediately 'fixed'

with fixing solution. This prevents the cells from drying out so that the laboratory can read the smear. The 'fixed' smear should be placed in a cool area and allowed to dry for 20 minutes.

The patient's details are written on the slide and the cervical cytology form must be completed. The slide is despatched to the **cytology** section of the pathology department for examination and reporting.

It is of vital importance that the patient is informed how she will obtain the results of the test. Patients should be informed in writing of any abnormal result or request for repeat of the test if an inadequate smear has been sent. **Deaths have occurred due to failure to follow this procedure.**

The following are some factors predisposing to cervical cancer:

- **Early age** at first intercourse.
- Many **sexual partners**.
- **Genital warts** (including those on partners).
- **Genital herpes**.
- **Smoking** - 20 cigarettes per day increases the risk by seven times.

Promiscuity is considered to be a factor as the more partners involved the more likely the causative factor (the wart virus is a strong suspect) may be encountered.

Positive results state findings such as:

- **dysplasia**   abnormal form
- **dyskaryosis**   abnormal nucleus
- **koilocytosis** having a spoon-shaped appearance, warty changes

Depending on the degree of abnormality of the cervical smear, the patient may be checked in six months or referred to the gynaecologist for a colposcopy and treatment.

Breast examination

Self-examination is still recommended for detection of this condition, but unfortunately if the lump can be felt the cancer is usually already well established. In the UK one in 12 women suffer from breast cancer at some time in their lives.

Mammography

This X-ray examination is recommended for women of **50 years to 64 years**. Prior to this the density of the breast tissue does not lend itself to satisfactory investigation by this method. Women over 64 years can also request a free test.

Regional Health Authorities have introduced

mass screening for women of the appropriate ages and a three-year **recall scheme** is in operation.

Testicular screening

Testicular screening is recommended for men, and routine manual examination of the scrotum is advised for detecting any abnormal development. Advances have been made in the treatment of this rapidly growing cancer.

Prostate cancer

For men with prostatism (enlargement of the prostate gland) a blood test for PSA (prostatic-specific antigen) will detect an increase in levels of this substance which may indicate the presence of carcinoma.

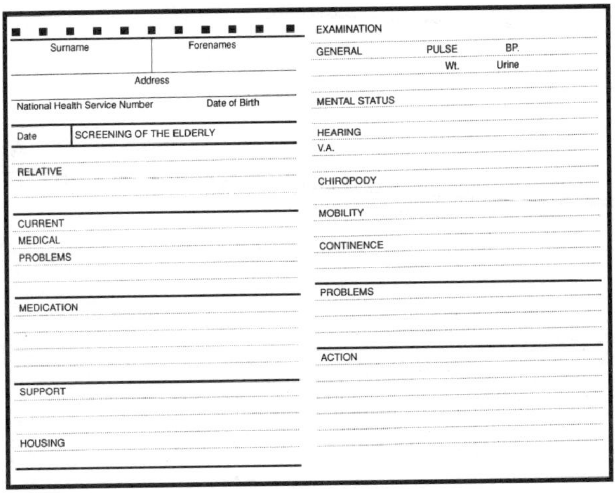
Surname | Forenames
Address
National Health Service Number | Date of Birth
Date | SCREENING OF THE ELDERLY
RELATIVE
CURRENT MEDICAL PROBLEMS
MEDICATION
SUPPORT
HOUSING
EXAMINATION
GENERAL PULSE BP. Wt. Urine
MENTAL STATUS
HEARING
V.A.
CHIROPODY
MOBILITY
CONTINENCE
PROBLEMS
ACTION

Figure 54 - Screening for the elderly card.

Cancer code

There is a 10-point European **cancer code** which aims to encourage people to live a healthy lifestyle to help avoid development of cancer. It includes:

- Stop smoking.
- Go easy on the alcohol - 21 units for men and 14 for women are the recommended weekly maximums, although these figures may be raised in the future.
- Avoid being overweight.
- Take care in the sun.
- Observe the Health and Safety at Work Regulations.
- Cut down on fatty foods.
- Eat plenty of fresh fruit and vegetables and other foods containing fibre.
- See your doctor if there is an unexplained change in your normal health which lasts for more than two weeks.

Cholesterol levels

A blood test for cholesterol levels is included in routine screening of at-risk adults. This is one of the fat components of the blood and is thought to be a factor in disease. A cholesterol above 5.2 mmol/l is considered an unnecessary risk. Diet is the first action to be taken. Levels should be checked in those with a family history of premature coronary disease and hypercholesterolaemia (high levels of cholesterol in the blood).

OTHER TESTS

There are many other conditions where screening would benefit the patient, including:

- **glaucoma**,
- **tuberculosis**,
- **large bowel cancer**,
- **diabetes mellitus,**
- **hypertension** (see Section 21).

HIV screening

The screening to detect antibodies to **human immunodeficiency virus** (HIV) is very carefully controlled. As there is no cure and the financial and social problems resulting are so devastating for the patient, **counselling must be given before any test is undertaken**.

Anonymous testing is being performed on blood taken from patients for other reasons. This is never associated back to the source and is purely to gain some knowledge of the spread of the disease.

New patient screening

This is a form of screening which is required under the 1990 Contract. Routine **testing of urine** and taking of **blood pressure** will often identify undetected health problems. Information on lifestyle and family history should identify at-risk individuals.

Screening of elderly people

Routine yearly screening of patients of **75 years and over** is also a requirement for GPs and various factors are assessed (Figure 54), including:

- **sensory function**,
- **mobility**,
- **mental condition**,
- **physical condition** including continence,
- **social environment**,
- **use of medicines**.

Elderly people are often suffering from the **side-effects of medication**, as with a reduced liver and kidney function due to the ageing process, smaller dosages may be required.

ABBREVIATIONS

CIN I-IV   cervical intra-epithelial neoplasia (classified according to the invasiveness of the neoplasm. CIN I denotes non-invasive)

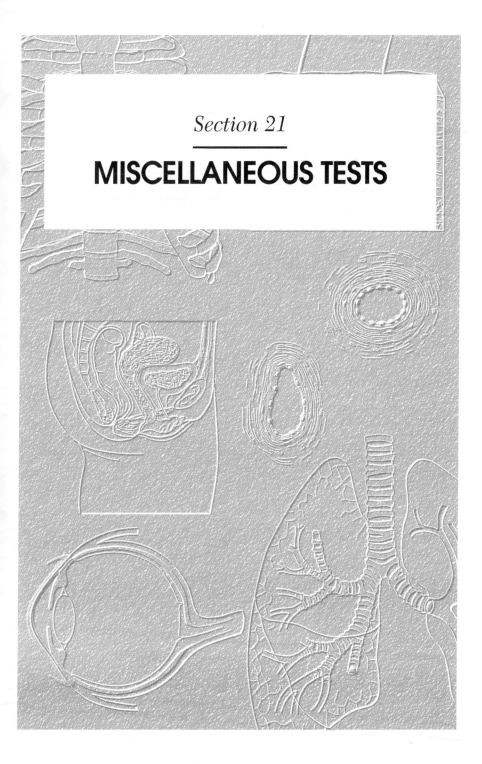

Section 21

MISCELLANEOUS TESTS

BLOOD PRESSURE MEASUREMENT

This is a common test used in general practice to measure arterial blood pressure. It reflects the state of the cardiac output and blood vessels. It is affected by age and illness (see Section 5).

The blood pressure is measured in millimeters of mercury (mmHg).

The **systolic pressure** is the pressure exerted against the walls of the arteries when the ventricles are contracting. The **diastolic pressure** is the pressure exerted on the walls of the arteries when the heart is relaxed. The condition of **hypertension** is diagnosed when the readings are abnormally high on three separate occasions.

Procedure

When using a **sphygmomanometer** a special cuff is applied to the arm of the patient, who should be lying or sitting and **be relaxed**. With patients who are on antihypertensive drugs, it should also be recorded with the patient standing.

A stethoscope is applied to the pulse of the **brachial artery** at the inner aspect of the elbow flexure. The cuff is inflated to obliterate the pulse and then the air in the cuff is slowly released. The pulse will return as a tapping sound. This will be the reading of the **systolic pressure**.

These sounds will continue but will then become fainter and rapidly diminish until they disappear. It will be at this point that the **diastolic pressure** will be interpreted.

In very low blood pressure (in severe shock) the systolic pressure may be obtained by **palpation** of the radial pulse. There will be no obtainable diastolic reading.

There are also meters which are now used to measure blood pressure automatically.

ELECTROCARDIOGRAPHY

An electrocardiogram (ECG) is a recording of the electrical impulses of the heart muscle as it beats. The apparatus transfers the impulses into a graph tracing so that they can be read and interpreted (see Figure 55). It is used to detect possible irregular rhythm and damage caused by myocardial infarct (coronary thrombosis). Most general practices have their own portable apparatus.

Tracings

The normal tracing of the heart is shown as the following:

The P-wave	illustrates the contraction of the atria.

The QRS complex	illustrates the conduction of the nerve impulse through the **bundle of His** in the ventricular septum of the heart into the ventricles.
The T-wave	illustrates the recovery of the ventricles.

Procedure

The leads, which are labelled for arms, legs and chest are placed on the patient, who must be at rest and lying on his/her back (see Figure 56). Special conducting jelly is applied to the plates attached and any excessive hair is removed with the patient's permission, by shaving. Any electrical interference must be eliminated; this may be from:

- wrist watch,
- other electrical apparatus,
- shivering of the patient if cold or apprehensive,
- main lead passing too close to the limb leads,
- nearby central heating radiator.

ELECTROENCEPHALOGRAPHY

An electroencephalogram (EEG) is used to detect abnormal electrical activity of the brain in the diagnosis of **epilepsy** and other lesions (abnormalities) such as **tumours of the brain**. The electrical activity is converted by the apparatus into a graph which can be read and interpreted.

Special conducting jelly is applied to the scalp and the leads attached. Differing areas are read and at one point lights are flashed to detect any abnormal response. Readings are taken with the patient's eyes closed and then open. The effect of hyperventilation (over-breathing) is also recorded.

Types of waves

These include **alpha**, **beta** and **theta** waves, the names given to the various types of electrical discharge from the brain.

EARLY MORNING URINE SPECIMEN (EMU)

This is a test for pregnancy. It is usually performed in the laboratory and the specimen collected must be a concentrated one, i.e. the first urine passed in the morning before drinking, and it must be uncontaminated by blood (in cases of

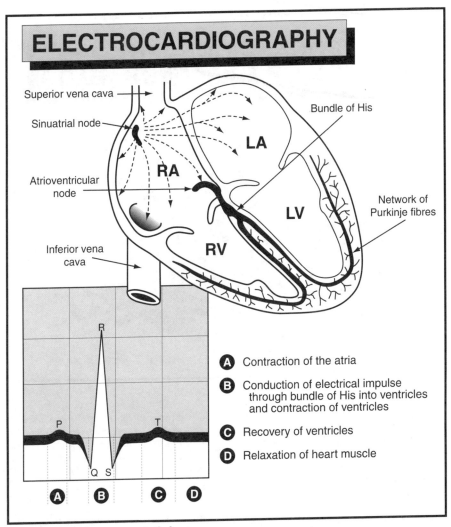

ELECTROCARDIOGRAPHY

Superior vena cava

Sinuatrial node

Atrioventricular node

Inferior vena cava

Bundle of His

LA

RA

LV

RV

Network of Purkinje fibres

R

P

T

Q S

A B C D

A Contraction of the atria

B Conduction of electrical impulse through bundle of His into ventricles and contraction of ventricles

C Recovery of ventricles

D Relaxation of heart muscle

Figure 55 - The conducting system in the heart.

threatened abortion etc.). If necessary a tampon must be inserted before the urine is passed.

The chemical test is based on the presence of **HCG** (human chorionic gonadotrophic hormone) present in the urine in pregnancy and verifies the presence of this chemical which is produced by the developing chorionic layer of the embryo.

A negative test does not necessarily signify that the patient is not pregnant. The test should be repeated. It is necessary for sufficient of the HCG to be present to give a positive result.

MIDSTREAM SPECIMEN OF URINE (MSU)

This test is performed to detect the presence of protein and micro-organisms in urine. **It is essential that the specimen is free from contamination by body fluids** which may be present on the external genitalia and it is for this reason that it is the middle part, or 'midstream', is used. The patient is requested to wash the external genitalia before passing the specimen. The first urine is passed in the normal way into the toilet, thus washing away any

ELECTROCARDIOGRAPHY POSITION OF THE CHEST LEADS

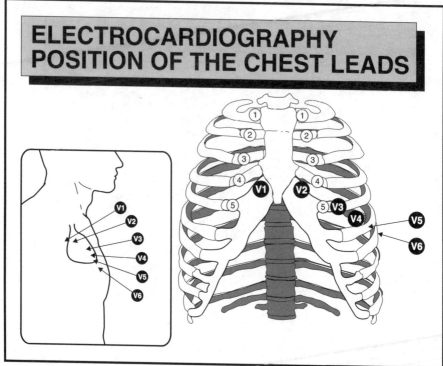

Figure 56 - Electrocardiography: position of the leads.

mucus present in the urethra. The next urine passed is received into the receptacle provided for the specimen, while the surplus urine is again passed into the toilet.

It is important that all specimens are immediately and correctly labelled to avoid any mistakes occurring. **Children or other vulnerable patients should never be left alone or given a glass receptacle for this test**. A suitable sterile jug or receiver should be used.

If the patient is to collect the specimen at home, a handout with full instructions on how to collect it is invaluable.

The specimen will usually be sent to the laboratory for culture and sensitivity (see Section 17).

ROUTINE URINE TESTING

This consists of testing for a variety of abnormalities.

Normal fresh urine is a sterile aromatic amber liquid with a specific gravity of 1.005 to 1.030 and a pH of five to seven (slightly acid).

The specific gravity will depend on the concentration of the urine. It can indicate disease of the

kidney and other conditions, e.g. diabetes insipidus.

Abnormal pH may indicate renal or other disease, but fever and diarrhoea will also affect this reading as well as the specific gravity.

Abnormal constituents tested for are:

Bile salts	present in certain types of jaundice.
Bilirubin	present in certain types of jaundice.
Blood	present in tumours of the bladder, cystitis, urethritis and kidney stones.
Glucose	present in diabetes mellitus and when taking certain drugs.
Ketones	(also known as **acetone**) - present when fats are inadequately burnt by body; present in diabetes mellitus imbalance **acidosis** and starvation states.

Nitrites	present in bacterial infection of the urine.
Phenylketones	present when the patient is unable to metabolise properly the nutrient phenylalanine. Accumulation of this in blood stream can cause mental retardation.
Protein	(usually albumin and blood) - present in infection, hypertension etc.
Urobilinogen	present in certain types of jaundice.

There are numerous **reagent test strips** on the market and it is vital that the urine is fresh and that the 'in-date' reagent strips are read at the correct time limits. **Instructions must be carefully followed, both for testing and storage of the components**.

BLOOD TESTS PERFORMED AT PRACTICE PREMISES

Many practices offer onsite blood testing as a fast service to patients, although these have decreased since concern of cross-infection from body fluids has been highlighted.

Glucose estimation

This determines the current levels present in blood. It is used for assisting in diagnosis of diabetes mellitus, routine monitoring of glucose levels and screening of patients where appropriate. Further laboratory tests are used to ensure accuracy. Reagent strips are used as in urine testing. There are also meters which measure content. Capillary blood is used, gathered from finger/heel prick as appropriate.

Cholesterol estimation

This is often offered as part of the 'well-person' check and can be used to back up dietary advice and assess patients response to diet or medication.

Other tests

Some surgeries offer the following tests:

Haemoglobin	measure of the oxygen-carrying capacity of the blood.
Erythrocite Sedimentation Rate (ESR)	rate at which red blood cells seperate from plasma.

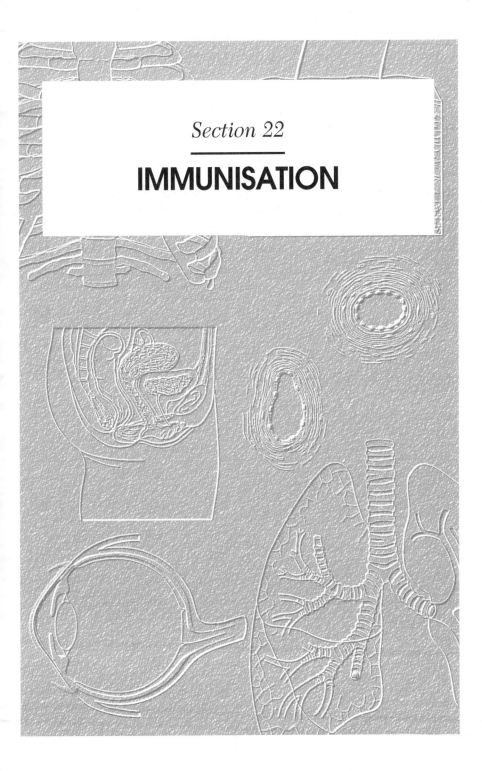

Section 22

IMMUNISATION

This is one of the most important areas of preventive medicine. It is concerned with the protection of the individual from specific diseases.

The first instance of it in the modern world, in the late 18th century, was by **Jenner** who vaccinated people with the cowpox virus to produce immunity against the killer virus of **smallpox**.

IMMUNITY

Immunity is the ability of the body to fight disease. It may be **natural** or **artificial**.

Natural immunity

Natural immunity is either an **inbuilt resistance** to a disease, e.g. human beings do not suffer from distemper found in dogs, or one that is 'acquired' by coming into contact with the actual disease and overcoming it.

Active immunity

This is a state in which the body has produced antibodies to a disease. It may be **natural** (by suffering an attack of the disease) or **artificial**, i.e. by introducing the weakened disease, or its poisons, into the body to allow the body to produce antibodies to the disease without suffering the harmful effects of the disease itself. This is the principle of immunisation.

Live viruses, such as the measles virus, are **attenuated** (weakened) so that they do not cause damage to the body but are still able to stimulate the body's immune system to produce antibodies against the virus.

Dead viruses, or bacteria, are also used in some vaccines as well as **weakened toxins**, e.g. diphtheria, tetanus and pertussis (whooping cough) vaccines.

Several doses at differing intervals usually have to be given to produce a sufficiently high level of **antibodies** to achieve immunity. This immunity will be **long-lasting** as the body has learnt how to produce the specific antibodies to the disease. It will immediately recognise the foreign protein of the disease should the person subsequently come into contact with it.

Passive immunity

This is achieved when **antibodies**, or **antitoxins**, produced by **another** person or animal are introduced into a person's body to fight disease. This immunity only lasts as long as the antibodies are present in the body, as the individual does **not** produce his/her own antibodies. Therefore this is only a **temporary immunity**, e.g. occurring naturally in **breast feeding** and

artificially when **immunoglobulin,** containing **hepatitis A** antibodies, is given to travellers, or susceptible people are given immunoglobulin against an attack of chicken-pox.

REASONS FOR IMMUNISATION

- to **protect** the individual,
- to **limit the spread** of a disease,
- to produce a '**herd**' immunity,
- to assist in **eradication** of the disease.

RECOMMENDED SCHEDULES

The Department of Health, through its Chief Medical Officer, recommends a **schedule** for children and travellers (see the 'Green Book' - *Immunisation against infectious disease, HMSO*). **Advice should always be sought from the Community Physician/Medical Officer when there is any query regarding suitablility and dosage for the individual patient.**

Below are the present recommendations for children and young persons:

2 months	**Hib**	1 injection
	DTP - diphtheria, tetanus and pertussis (whooping cough)	Combined Vaccine
	poliomyelitis	by mouth
3 months	**Hib**	1 injection
	DTP	Combined Vaccine
	poliomyelitis	by mouth
4 months	**Hib**	1 injection
	DTP	Combined Vaccine
	poliomyelitis	by mouth
At 12 - 15 months	**measles, mumps and rubella (MMR)**	1 injection Combined Vaccine
3 - 5 years (usually prior to school entry)	**diphtheria, tetanus (DT)**	1 booster injection
	poliomyelitis	booster by mouth
	MMR	second dose injection
10 - 14 years (sometimes shortly after birth)	**turberculosis**	1 injection after skin testing e.g
	BCG	Heaf or Mantoux tests

School leavers 13 - 18 years	diphtheria, tetanus Td (low-dose diphtheria)	1 booster injection
	poliomyelitis	booster by mouth

RELEVANT CHILDHOOD DISEASES

Diphtheria

This acute upper respiratory disease, caused by bacteria, is unfortunately increasing in its occurrence after being well-controlled in routine immunisation of children. The toxins produced by the causative organism *Corynebacteria diphtheriae* can cause damage to the heart and nervous system. It can also cause an acute and rapid onset in difficulty in breathing as a result of the production of a greyish membrane in the airway, causing death in severe cases. It is an **airborne** disease usually spread by droplet infection and contact with **fomites** (objects contaminated by an infected person). The vaccine is composed of **weakened** toxins.

Tetanus

Tetanus is caused by **contact** with the bacteria *Tetanus bacillus* which is commonly found in soil. The organism is capable of producing protective spores which enable it to survive in anaerobic (without air) conditions. Entrance to the body may be through cuts, burns or scratches from roses. In Third World countries such as Africa and Asia the newborn baby's umbilical stump may become infected. It is not transmitted from person to person. The toxins produced by the bacteria may cause spasms and paralysis, and the inability to breath can cause death if treatment is delayed; emergency tracheostomy (artificial opening into the windpipe) is used to treat this complication. The vaccine is composed of **weakened toxins**.

Pertussis (whooping cough)

Pertussis is a killer disease and in unimmunised children produces prolonged coughing spasms and a characteristic 'whoop' as air rushes into the airway as a spasm ceases. The toxins produced by the bacteria cause vomiting and periods of **apnoea** (absence of breathing), and death from choking and other complications (e.g. **bronchopneumonia**) is common in children under 6 months of age. This highly infectious **airborne** disease, caused by the bacteria *Bordetella pertussis*, is spread by **droplet** infection. The vaccine is composed of **dead** bacteria.

Hib (Haemophilus influenzae type B) and meningitis

Hib causes serious illnesses, such as meningitis, pneumonia, epiglottitis and other problems in young children. The vaccine is mainly given to prevent meningitis, but is only active against the specific infection caused by Hib and does not prevent **meningitis** caused by other organisms, e.g. **meningococcal** meningitis and **viral** meningitis. The disease is **airborne**, spread by **droplet** infection. Incidence of the disease, usually found in children under 1 year, has dropped dramatically since the introduction of the Hib vaccine schedule. The vaccine does **not** consist of live organisms.

The early signs and symptoms of meningitis are headache, fever, irritability, restlessness, vomiting and refusal of feeds (common with the symptoms of other illnesses such as colds and

---

BOX 1 – MENINGITIS: *what to look for*

In babies look for the following:

- A high-pitched, moaning cry.
- The child being difficult to wake.
- Refusing to feed.
- Pale or blotchy skin.
- Red or purple spots that do not fade under pressure – do the 'Glass Test' (see below)

In older children look for the following signs:

- Red or purple spots that do not fade under pressure.
- Stiffness in the neck – can the child kiss his or her knee, or touch his or her forehead to the knee?
- Drowsiness or confusion.
- A severe headache.
- A dislike of bright light.

The 'Glass Test'. Press the side of a glass firmly against the rash – you will be able to see it if it fades and loses colour under the pressure. If it doesn't change colour, contact your doctor immediately.

If your child becomes ill with one or more of these symptoms and signs, contact your doctor urgently. You may be asked to go straight to the surgery.

If your child has a rash of red or purple spots or bruises, get medical help immediately.

Source: Health Education Authority (1997) A *Guide to Childhood Immunisation*, 19

181

influenza). Babies can become seriously ill within hours; the presence of a high-pitched, moaning cry together with drowsiness are both signs. In older children, dislike of light and neck rigidity are warning signs. The presence of a red or purple skin rash, **which does not fade under pressure**, indicates **septicaemia**. Advice can be obtained from the leaflet *A Guide to Childhood Immunisations* produced by the Health Education Authority (Box 1), which also provides specific advice on what to look for in babies and children and how to act accordingly.

Poliomyelitis

Polio is caused by a viral infection which, following invasion of the gastrointestinal tract, attacks the grey matter in the **central nervous system**. Spread via **water** and **faeces**, it can cause paralysis and death from the inability to breath. **The faeces passed by the recently immunised child or person can cause the illness to develop in an unprotected person**. Baby carers who change the immunised child's nappies should ensure that they are properly protected and immunised. For this reason, booster doses of oral polio are often given to parents at the same time as their children are immunised. Poliomyelitis remains **endemic** in many Third World countries and in industrialised countries such as the UK there are sporadic outbreaks, usually associated with unimmunised individuals. The **oral** vaccine consists of a 'live' attenuated (weakened) virus.

Measles

Measles is highly infectious and can kill, so it is important that routine immunisation is given. General malaise, coryza (runny nose) and headache herald the beginning of the infection. On approximately the fourth day of the disease a distinctive skin rash appears consisting of **macules. Koplik spots** in the mouth may be apparent prior to the skin rash and will determine a differential diagnosis of this condition. Measles occurs due to an **airborne** virus which can cause high fever, otitis media (inflammation of the middle ear), conjunctivitis, convulsions, respiratory infection such as bronchopneumonia, and brain damage. The vaccine given is a 'live' attenuated preparation.

Mumps

Mumps is an **airborne**, viral infection and causes inflammation and swelling of the salivary glands, especially the parotid glands. Complications can cause deafness, pancreatitis (inflammation of the pancreas) and swelling of the testicles and ovaries, which may result in **sterility**. Spread by **droplet infection**, mumps may also inflame the brain, causing meningitis and encephalitis. The vaccine contains a 'live' attenuated virus.

Rubella

Rubella (commonly known as German measles) is caused by an **airborne** virus spread by **droplet infection**. It usually produces a mild illness characterised by a fleeting rash similar to measles and a fever. Serological investigation, where indicated, is required for proof of the infection as many diseases produce a similar skin rash. However, if a woman catches the disease in **early pregnancy, deformity** of the developing fetus is common. Damage may also be done if the woman is not aware that she is pregnant.

The routine immunisation of girls in their early teens has now been replaced with the routine MMR immunisation of all children at an earlier age. The vaccine is a **live** attenuated one.

Tuberculosis

Tuberculosis is caused by an infection with bacteria (e.g. *Myobacterium tuberculosis*). It is an **airborne** infection which is easily spread by **droplet** infection. Infection of the lungs is the most common form of the disease, but other organs can become infected as a result of drinking milk from infected animals, particularly in Third World countries. Unfortunately, drug resistant strains have emerged and are **increasing** worldwide. Despite the increase in reported cases, the disease is relatively rare in the UK.

BCG (Bacillus Calmette-Guérin) vaccine

BCG is a 'live' attenuated vaccine given to protect against tuberculosis. A routine skin test (**Heaf or Mantoux test**) is performed on the arm by introducing dead tuberculin bacilli intradermally in order to determine the person's antibody levels to tuberculosis. If the person has been exposed to the disease, the results of the skin test will show a **positive** reaction. The vaccine will **not** be given if the skin test is positive. Cases of positive reaction will be **screened** for active tuberculosis.

Varicella (chickenpox)

Varicella is a highly infectious disease caused by a virus. Papules, vesicles and subsequently pustules appear on the face and scalp, spreading to the trunk, abdomen and limbs. The major distribution is towards the centre of the body surface, and lesions also occur on the mucous membranes of the respiratory tract. The three stages of skin eruption will be present as successive crops of papules arise throughout the course of the disease. Eventually all lesions will dry up and the scabs will be shed. The disease is spread by **droplet** infection, personal **contact**, and **fomites**. **Shingles (herpes zoster)** is a condition in which the varicella virus is reactivated in the body of an individual who has previously recovered from a case of chickenpox. At present there is no active vaccine available in this country, but a **'live' attenuated** one is licenced in other countries such as the **USA**.

ADULT IMMUNISATION

Recommended **booster** immunisations for adults are for **tetanus** and **poliomyelitis**. It is advisable to check the immunisation status of all **new** patients. The continued coverage of protection against **diphtheria** is vital to stop the disease **recurring** in this country.

Tetanus

At present a booster dose is recommended every 10 years (previously five years). **Checking of current status is important for all new patients**.

Poliomyelitis

Adults under the age of 40 years should receive boosters every 10 years if travelling outside the UK, and parents should receive boosters at the same time as their baby commences immunisation.

Diphtheria

A **low-dose vaccine** is available for those individuals over the age of 10 years. Primary immunisation is indicated for all adults not previously protected. (The old Schick test for susceptibility to the disease is now no longer used.)

CONTRAINDICATIONS TO IMMUNISATION

Each case must be looked at individually by the physician responsible for administering the vaccine. The following should be considered:

- if the child is **unwell** or has a **fever**.

1. YOUR TRAVEL VACCINE RECORD

✓ Visit your surgery well in advance as some vaccines need to be given a month or more before you go.

✓ Remember that for some vaccines, to ensure long-term protection, you will need to come back for a booster vaccination.

Vaccine		Date received	Booster due date
Hepatitis A	Primary		
	First Booster		
Typhoid			
Meningococcal A+C			
Yellow Fever			
Diphtheria/Tetanus			
Tetanus			
Polio			

Continued on inside back cover

1. YOUR TRAVEL VACCINE RECORD (cont.)

Vaccine		Date received	Booster due date
Japanese Enc	Dose 1		
	Dose 2		
	(Dose 3)		
Tick-borne encephalitis			
Rabies	Dose 1		
	Dose 2		
	Dose 3		
Hepatitis B	Dose 1		
	Dose 2		
	Dose 3		
	(Dose 4)		
Other			
Malaria		Remember to ask you doctor/nurse/pharmacist for advice where appropriate	

Figure 57 - Immunisation record card. Reproduced with kind permission from Pasteur Mérieux MSD Ltd.

- if the child has had a **reaction to previous immunisations**.
- if the child has had previous **severe allergic reaction to eating eggs**.
- if the child is taking **medicines** for other conditions (**especially steroids**), is immunodeficient, or has recently received passive immunisation of immunoglobulin.

If the child suffers from **fits** or there is a close **family history**, the doctor will discuss and review any likely problem with the parent. Stable neurological conditions may not indicate contraindication.

Contraindications for adults are similar, but **pregnancy** is included as any immunisation may damage the fetus.

When live vaccines are to be given, special consideration of risks must be made in order to ensure the patient's immune response is not impaired because of any already existing condition or disease. **Certain live vaccines must not be given within a fixed period of each other.**

CONSENT

Consent from the parent for children under 16 years is normally essential and there should be a **protocol** to be followed for children accompanied by someone other than the parent. **This is extremely important from a legal aspect.** Written consent is not essential but provides permanent **proof** of agreement should future problems arise. Consent is required for **each** immunisation given.

Any likely side-effect etc., must be discussed by the doctor with the parent before consent is given. **It should be noted** that a young person under 16 years of age may give or refuse consent for immunisation or treatment provided that he/she **understands fully** the benefits and risks involved. Whether giving or refusing consent, the child should always be encouraged to involve the parent or guardian in the decision. **Immunisation should not be given against the young person's wishes.**

VACCINE DAMAGE PAYMENTS

Unfortunately, a few children suffer damage as a result of immunisation. There is now a single tax-free payment for people who have suffered severe mental and/or physical **disablement** of 80% or more as a result of immunisation against one or more of the following diseases:

- Diphtheria
- Tetanus
- Pertussis
- Poliomyelitis
- Rubella
- Measles
- Tuberculosis
- Mumps
- Smallpox
- *Haemophilus influenzae* type b (Hib)

There is a time and age limitation to this compensation award.

REPORTING OF ADVERSE REACTIONS

Any adverse reaction to immunisation should be reported on the 'yellow card' system and sent to the Medical Control Agency (MCA). Information should include **vaccine** and **batch numbers,** which will alert the authority to any general problems arising and so prevent further damage (as seen in the '**thalidomide**' disaster when a drug was prescribed to women in the first trimester of pregnancy which resulted in children being born with varying degrees of deformity, especially the presence of only rudimentary limbs). Evidence is considered by the **Joint Committee on Vaccination and Immunisation** (JCVI), an independent body providing expert advice on policy, safety and efficacy of vaccines.

Reporting for doctors is voluntary, but is a **statutory** requirement for drug companies and vaccine manufacturers.

TARGETS

At present the HA conditions under the 1990 Contract require **90%** of children under five years to be immunised for diphtheria, tetanus, pertussis, poliomyelitis and Hib to achieve the higher target payment and **70%** to receive the lower payment.

ROLE OF RECEPTIONIST

The receptionist will be involved in recall and records of children for immunisation. It is important that all data are **properly** recorded and notes are properly filed (see Figure 57).

The **immediate reporting** to the doctor or nurse, of any information that may have been told to the receptionist by the parent, concerning a baby's reaction to a previous immunisation or fears concerning a particular injection, such as pertussis, is most important. This can avoid prob-

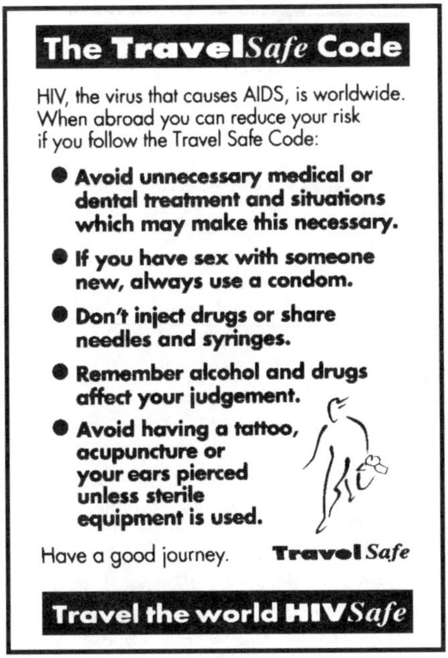

Figure 58 - The travelsafe code card (source: HEA).

lems as often these fears are not repeated to the person administering the vaccine.

The **provision** of current health education leaflets and posters is also an important requirement.

It is also important that the receptionist is aware of the need to be alert to patients who visit the doctor following **recent return from abroad**. If illness occurs within three weeks, it is necessary to isolate the patient from other patients in the waiting room in order to avoid cross-infection. **Until the patient has been diagnosed s/he must be considered a health risk to others**.

BATCH NUMBERS AND EXPIRY DATES

These are recorded on the special forms by the person giving the injection and **records** must be kept in case of any reaction.

STORAGE

Vaccines must be kept at the correct temperature as stated on the bottle and in the literature. **A refrigerator, other than the one used for food and milk etc., must be kept for this purpose and temperature levels must be** **carefully checked**; a temperature of between 2 and 8°C is the usual requirement, although some polio vaccines require storage at 0–4°C. The contents and strength of the vaccine will be adversely affected if it is incorrectly stored.

The temperature should never be allowed to sink below 0°C, as freezing can damage the efficacy of the vaccine and also break the container.

Position in the refrigerator is also important; shelves or compartments in the **door** must **never** be used. Specialist refrigerators designed for medicine and vaccines are obtainable.

Maximum and minimum temperatures should be recorded regularly, preferably daily. Written procedures should be provided and, if the temperature requirements are breached, necessary reporting to the appropriate person. There should be clear designated responsibility for both monitoring and reporting.

Arrangements for cold storage must be made to allow regular defrosting of refrigerators if an alternative one is not available.

Transportation of vaccines

Transportation of vaccines must be carefully monitored to ensure damage to their content does not occur. Temperature control must be maintained and monitored throughout the period of transportation.

If vaccines have been sent by post, they should not be accepted if more than 48 hours have elapsed since the time of despatch. First-class post must be used and all necessary instructions regarding the materials and hazards should be followed.

Disposal

Great care must be taken to ensure safe disposal of empty or unused, expired vials by **incineration** or **heat inactivation**. The requirements of the **Environmental Protection Act 1990** and regulations governing the disposal of **clinical waste** must be strictly followed and written procedures should be provided. Disposal in the **'sharps' bin** followed by incineration is usually the required procedure in general practice. Information and advice may be obtained from the local consultant in Communicable Disease Control.

TRAVELLERS

Travellers require special protection according to the area in which they are to be travelling. Information and advice is available to doctors from the **Communicable Disease**

Surveillance Centre. The newspaper *PULSE* issues monthly bulletins on these requirements. This is based on recommendations issued from the **World Health Organisation**.

Recommended schedule for travellers

As well as the following schedule for travellers, a recent special health education card produced by the Health Education Authority with advice on preventing HIV risk is shown in Figure 58. Travellers to remote areas or Third World countries are also advised to carry a **sterile set of basic dental and surgical requirements,** including an intravenous 'giving set'. The reuse of injection needles is a common occurrence in these areas, and travellers have been **cross-infected** with Hepatitis B and HIV. Hepatitis C is also a hazard and at present there is no vaccine available. **Hepatitis B** is far more virulent than **HIV**; it is not killed by boiling the equipment and requires strict **autoclaving procedures** for its elimination.

All travellers are recommended for immunisation against diphtheria, poliomyelitis and tetanus if not previously immunised.

All areas **except** North and West Europe, North America, Australia and New Zealand	**poliomyelitis**
All areas with poor standards of hygiene and sanitation	**typhoid and hepatitis A**
Infected areas as advised	**anti-malaria tablets, precautions against mosquitoes, yellow fever, tuberculosis**
In some circumstances	**diphtheria, hepatitis B, rabies, Japanese encephalitis, tick encephalitis, meningococcal meningitis**

International certificates

These are internationally recognised certificates verifying that the named person has received immunisation against a particular disease. They are available for **yellow fever,** but **not** for cholera as people do not require immunisation against it. **At present, a signed medical state-ment to this effect can be issued to those travelling to an epidemic area.**

International certificates are signed by the doctor responsible for administering the vaccine. It is **compulsory** to have an international certificate for entry to some countries.

The special vaccines available for travellers are:

Yellow fever

This is a live vaccine and is only available from **special centres.** Special storage is required. An initial immunisation is followed by booster injection every 10 years.

Cholera

Currently, there is **no vaccine** available in this country. However, an oral vaccine is being developed which will hopefully prove more efficient than previous ones.

Typhoid

There are three vaccines available at present; two for injection and one 'live' attenuated oral preparation. Requirements of **dosage** and **boosters vary** according to the preparation used. The current recommended final boosters are required at **3-year intervals,** however manufacturer's suggestions should be followed. Immunity to paratyphoid infection is not provided.

Smallpox

This is now no longer required as the disease has been eradicated.

Hepatitis A

This is advised for visitors to Third World countries or areas where sanitation is poor. **Until recently** this has been a **passive form** of immunisation provided by the administration of human immunoglobulin containing antibodies to the disease. Immunisation must be given immediately before departure and protection lasts approximately 3 months. However, there is now an **active immunisation** available, which is preferable.

The single protection vaccines for hepatitis A active immunity advise booster doses every 10 years following the initial schedule. Manufacturer's recommendations vary according to the product.

Hepatitis A and B

There is now a combined vaccine available for both hepatitis A and B which, following the administration of the initial recommended schedule, gives protection for 5 years. Antibody levels must be measured to ensure protection.

Three injections are required; two within a month and a third injection 6 months later. Antibody levels must be checked to ensure successful immunisation. Booster doses are required at **3- to 5-yearly** intervals according to levels of antibody titre.

Poliomyelitis

This immunisation should be given to travellers to third-world countries where **hygiene** is primitive. A booster dose is required every **10 years.**

Tetanus

This is recommended for **all** travellers if their present immunisation against tetanus is not up to date. A **10-yearly** booster is recommended.

Diphtheria

Those previously covered by routine immunisations should be offered **low-dose** immunisation every **10–20 years.** Travellers to Russia and certain eastern European countries where the disease is **endemic** should be offered boosters. (**Primary** immunisation is indicated for individuals who have **never received** immunisation for this disease.)

Meningococcal Meningitis

This is a vaccine available to protect travellers against certain strains of this bacterial infection. Travellers to **sub-Saharan** areas of **Africa** are advised to be immunised with this vaccine.

Malaria

Travellers to declared areas of known malarial risk should be advised to take **precautions** to avoid this disease. The **mosquito** is the carrier for this disease and it is prevalent in tropical and subtropical areas over a wide area, e.g. **India and Africa.**

Unfortunately, due to mosquitoes entering **aeroplanes**, it is also possible to contract malaria from airports en route, where the disease of malaria would not be expected. There have even been cases thought to have been contracted in this way close to **Gatwick Airport** in England.

The sharing of infected needles is also a means of infection. Advice concerning prevention of mosquito bites must be given. **Special tablets must be started at least a week before departure and continued for a period of one month following return.**

Unfortunately, resistance is increasing to many forms of treatments and the drug given will depend upon the **area to be visited.**

Japanese B Encephalitis

This vaccine may be offered to those travellers residing in **south-east Asia** for **1 month** or more. It is a viral infection and the vaccine is composed of a **killed** virus.

Other immunisations available

Other immunisations available include those against **influenza, pneumococcal disease** and **hepatitis B.** Vaccines are also available against **anthrax** for those workers at risk and **rabies** (hydrophobia) for those persons who may have been bitten by a rabid animal.

Influenza

This is commonly given to patients 'at risk', i.e. **elderly** people, patients with **asthma** and those with other **chronic respiratory or cardiovascular disease**. It is usual to have campaigns alerting patients to protect themselves against the yearly epidemics which occur. Booster doses are given yearly and the vaccine is developed wherever possible to combat the particular strain of the virus. Special fees are payable at present from HAs.

Pneumococcal Infections

This vaccine is offered routinely to those at risk from bacterial respiratory infections. Patients recommended for this vaccine include those with **immunodeficiency, diabetes mellitus, chronic liver, lung and heart disease**, and individuals who have had their **spleen removed**. One dose is given and booster doses are **not** normally administered.

Hepatitis B

This active immunisation is available for those at risk, whether due to their lifestyle or occupation. **Practice staff who are likely to come into contact with body fluids from infected persons need to be protected (a requirement under regulations of the Health and Safety at Work).** It is not always known who is infected with this virus as the incubation period can be up to **6 months** and **carriers** have no symptoms.

Three injections are required; two within a month and a third injection 6 months later. Antibody levels must be checked to ensure successful immunisation. Booster doses are required at **3- to 5-yearly intervals**, according to levels of antibody titre.

There are different varieties of vaccine and manufacturer's recommendations must be followed.

A **passive immunisation** of a specific immunoglobulin (Hepatitis B immune globulin) is also available for immediate temporary protection in cases of accidental inoculation, 'needle-stick' injuries, or contamination with antigen-positive blood. This specific passive immunity does not affect the development of active immunity, so combined passive/active immunisation is recommended in certain cases of post-exposure treatment.

Anaphylactic Shock

There is always the risk of a patient being administered a vaccine and developing anaphylactic shock. This **potentially fatal condition,** occurring in response to the administration of a foreign protein, can happen rapidly without any warning, producing a variety of clinical features, ranging from respiratory difficulties to immediate cardiovascular collapse and death. Signs may include **skin rash, noisy breathing** due to **bronchospasm** and **oedema**, and loss of consciousness. **Immediate resuscitation techniques must be available and life-support drugs such as adrenalin must always be available whenever immunisation is being performed.** Guidelines are available from the Department of Health and the local community physician/medical officer.

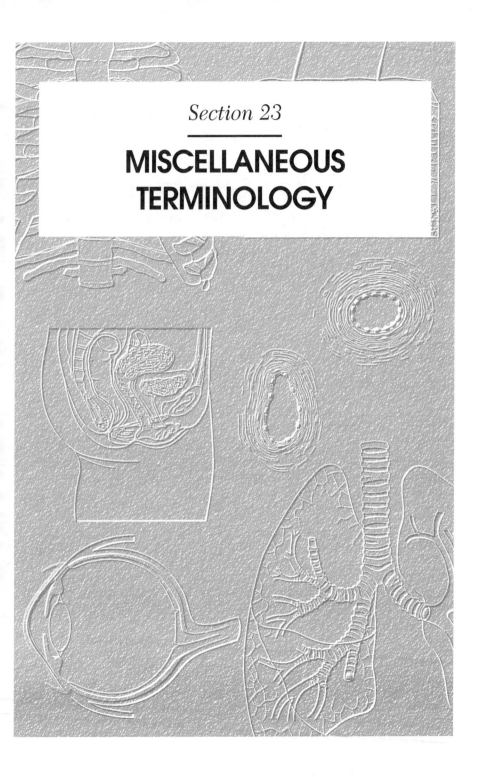

Section 23

MISCELLANEOUS TERMINOLOGY

TERMINOLOGY OF MEDICAL SPECIALITIES

Anaesthesia (anaesthetist) concerning the administration of anaesthetics.

Cardiology (cardiologist) concerning the heart and blood vessels.

Dermatology (dermatologist) concerning skin.

Endocrinology (endocrinologist) concerning the endocrine system.

Gastroenterology (gastroenterologist) concerning the digestive system.

Genitourinary (genitourinary physician) concerning the urinary system and male reproductive system.

Gerontology (geriatrician) concerning disorders of elderly people.

Gynaecology (gynaecologist) concerning the female reproductive system.

Haematology (haematologist) concerning the blood.

Immunology (immunologist) concerning immunity (defence of the body).

Nephrology (nephrologist) concerning the urinary system.

Neurology (neurologist) concerning the nervous system.

Obstetrics (obstetrician) concerning pregnancy and childbirth.

Ophthalmology (ophthalmologist) concerning eye disease.

Orthopaedics (orthopaedic surgeon) concerning disorders of the locomotor system.

Otorhinolaryngology (ENT surgeon) concerning ear, nose and throat disorders.

Paediatrics (paediatrician) concerning children's diseases.

Pathology (pathologist) concerning diagnosis of disease and examination of patient samples and dead bodies by post-mortem.

Forensic pathology criminal investigation.

Physician concerning medical conditions (as opposed to surgical).

Psychiatry (psychiatrist) concerning mental illness.

Radiology (radiologist) concerning use of X-rays in diagnosis and treatment.

Rheumatology (rheumatologist) concerning disease and conditions of connective tissue.

Surgery (surgeon) concerning surgery (as opposed to medical treatment).

Urology (Urologist) concerning the urinary system.

Venereology (venereologist) concerning sexually transmitted diseases.

Non-medical specialities

Audiometry (audiometrist) concerned with the measurement of hearing.

Optometry (optician) concerning the measurement of refraction (ability to focus) of the eye and dispensing spectacles.

Orthodontistry (orthodontist) concerning correction of teeth (dentition).

Orthoptics (orthoptist) treatment and diagnosis of squints etc.

Physiotherapy (physiotherapist) concerning treatment by physical exercise etc.

Psychology (psychologist) concerning behaviour including the normal.

Radiography (radiographer) concerning the taking of X-rays and delivery of treatment.

CLASSIFICATION OF DISEASES AND ASSOCIATED TERMS

Acquired occurring after birth.

Acute of sudden onset.

Aetiology the scientific study of the cause of disease.

Allergic hypersensitivity to foreign protein.

Atrophy wastage or shrinking of an organ.

Benign not malignant - has a good prognosis.

Chronic of long, slow duration.

Congenital present at birth.

Diagnosis decision of what is wrong with the patient by considering signs and symptoms.

Differential diagnosis One of a list of possible diagnoses, given the signs and symptoms prented, e.g. differential diagnoses of chest pains include indigestion, myocardial infarction etc.

Dystrophy	abnormal nourishment or function of an organ.
Empirical	treatment that is given because it works although there is no known scientific reason why it does.
Epidemiology	study of the cause of disease including social factors.
Exacerbate	make worse.
Functional	effects the body function.
Hypertrophy	excessive growth or development of an organ with its own tissue.
Iatrogenic	condition caused by the doctor, usually by side-effects of medication.
Idiopathic	of unknown origin.
Infective(ious)	a disease capable of being spread from one person to others.
Malignant	harmful, damaging, e.g. cancer.
Metabolic	concerning the basic working or metabolism of the body.
Morbid	abnormal.
Neoplastic	producing new growths, i.e. cancerous.
Organic	effects the structure of the body.
Prognosis	the forecast of the probable course and outcome of a disease.
Sub-clinical	not producing any obvious signs or symptoms.
Syndrome	a collection of three or more signs and symptoms which together form a disease, e.g. Down's syndrome.
Systemic	widespread/throughout the body.
Toxic	caused by poisons - poisonous.
Traumatic	caused by injury/ damage.

MISCELLANEOUS ABBREVIATIONS

A&E	accident and emergency
AET	aged
ARC	AIDS-related complex
BID	brought in dead
BP	blood pressure
BS	breath sounds
Ca	carcinoma/calcium
CO C/O	complains of (or carbon monoxide)
Cx	cervix
Dec	deceased
DNA	did not attend/ deoxyribonucleic acid
DNR	do not resuscitate
DOA	dead on arrival
DOB/dob	date of birth
Dxr	deep X-ray
ENT	ear, nose and throat
ESN	educationally sub-normal
FH	family history/fetal heart
FNA	fine needle aspiration (for cytology investigation)
GOK	god only knows
HDU	high dependency unit
H/O	history of
Hx	history
IA, i.a.	intra-articular
ICU	intensive care unit
IgA	immunoglogulin (gamma) A
IgBF	immunoglobulin (gamma) binding factor
IgD	immunoglobulin (gamma) D
IgE	immunoglobulin (gamma) E
IgG	immunoglobulin (gamma) G
IgM	immunoglobulin (gamma) M
IM, i.m.	intramuscular
IP	inpatient
IQ	intelligence quotient

IM, i.m.	intramuscular	**TCI**	to come in
IP	inpatient	**TLC**	tender loving care
IQ	intelligence quotient	**TPR**	temperature, pulse and respirations
ISQ	in status quo (no change)	**TTA**	to take away
IT	intrathecal	**UPLD**	upper limb disorder
ITU	intensive therapy unit	**WRULD**	work related upper limb disorder
IV, i.v.	intravenous		
NAD	no abnormality detected/demonstrated	**YOB**	year of birth

IM, i.m. intramuscular
IP inpatient
IQ intelligence quotient
ISQ in status quo (no change)
IT intrathecal
ITU intensive therapy unit
IV, i.v. intravenous
NAD no abnormality detected/demonstrated
NG new growth (neoplasm)
NOAD no other abnormality detected
OA on arrival/osteoarthritis
OE on examination
OP outpatient
OPD outpatient department
PCO patient complains of
PH past history
PMH past medical history
POP plaster of Paris
PP private patient
PR per rectum (rectal examination)
PUO pyrexia of unknown origin
PV per vaginam
RSI repetitive strain injury
RTA road traffic accident
SMI school medical inspection
SOB shortness of breath
Sx surgery, suction, symptoms and signs
TATT tired all the time
TCA to come again

TCI to come in
TLC tender loving care
TPR temperature, pulse and respirations
TTA to take away
UPLD upper limb disorder
WRULD work related upper limb disorder
YOB year of birth

SIGNS

Δ diagnosis
ΔΔ differential diagnoses
> greater than
< less than
+ve positive
-ve negative
↑/↓ increase/decrease
℞ recipe/take
c. with
s. without
3/7 three days
1/52 one week
1/12 one month
°jaundice no jaundice
°oedema no oedema
fracture
μg microgram
↔ or N normal
Ψ psychiatric
♀ female
♂ male
† deceased
* birth
⚢ female homosexual
⚣ male homosexual

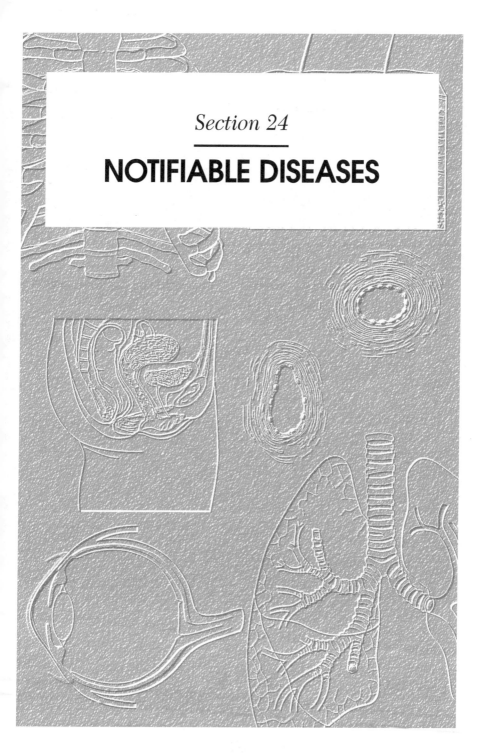

Section 24

NOTIFIABLE DISEASES

Certain infectious illnesses and food poisoning are reportable (Table 12). In England and Wales this is governed by:

- **The Public Health (Control of Diseases) Act 1984.**
- **The Public Health (Infectious Diseases) Regulations 1968 and 1985 (concerning AIDS) and various other regulations.**

In Scotland the following legislation applies:

- **Infectious Diseases (Notification Act 1889).**
- **Public Health (Scotland) Act 1897.**
- **Food and Drugs (Scotland) Act 1957.**

If the medical practitioner considers or suspects that a patient is suffering from a notifiable disease, it is a legal requirement to immediately inform the **'proper officer'**. The proper officer is usually, but not always, the Medical Officer of the Environmental Health Department of the Local Authority. Similarly, in Scotland it may be the Chief Administrative Medical Officer to the Health Board.

Doctors are **paid a nominal fee** for the notification, and special forms are provided by the Public Health Department for this purpose. The certificate (completed by the attending physician) is normally the means of notification and requires information on the patient's:

Table 12 – Notifiable Diseases

England and Wales	Northern Ireland	Scotland
Acute encephalitis	Acute encephalitis/	Anthrax
Acute poliomyelitis	meningitis: bacterial	Chickenpox
Anthrax	Acute encephalitis/	Cholera
Cholera	meningitis: viral	Diphtheria
Diphtheria	Anthrax	Dysentery
Dysentery (amoebic	Chickenpox	(bacillary)
or bacillary)	Cholera	Erysipelas
Food poisoning (all sources)	Diphtheria	Food poisoning
Leprosy	Dysentery	Legionellosis
Leptospirosis	Food poisoning	Lyme disease
Malaria	Gastroenteritis	Measles
Measles	(persons under two years	Membranous croup
Meningitis	of age only)	Meningococcal
Meningococcal septicaemia	Hepatitis	infection
(without meningitis)	A Hepatitis	Mumps
Mumps	B Hepatitis	Paratyphoid fever
Opthalmia neonatorum	unspecified: viral	Plague
Paratyphoid fever	Legionnaire's disease	Poliomyelitis
Plague	Leptospirosis	Puerperal fever
Rabies	Malaria	Rabies
Relapsing fever	Measles	Relapsing fever
Rubella	Meningococcal septicaemia	Rubella

Scarlet fever	Mumps	Scarlet fever
Smallpox	Paratyphoid fever	Smallpox
Tetanus	Plague	Tetanus
Tuberculosis	Poliomyelitis: acute	Toxoplasmosis
Typhoid fever	Rabies	Tuberculosis
Typhus	Relapsing fever	Typhoid fever
Viral haemorrhagic fevers	Rubella	Typhus
Viral hepatitis	Scarlet fever	Viral haemorrhagic
Whooping cough	Smallpox	fevers
Yellow fever	Tetanus	Viral hepatitis
	Tuberculosis: pulmonary and non-pulmonary	Whooping cough
	Typhoid fever	
	Typhus	
	Viral haemorrhagic fevers	
	Whooping cough	Source: *The Medical Protection Society (1988).*
	Yellow fever	

Although smallpox disease has been eliminated, it remains a notifiable disease.

- **Name.**
- **Address.**
- **Sex and age.**
- **Name of the disease.**
- **Date of the onset of the illness.**

If the patient is in hospital, then further details are required, including:

- The **address** from which the patient was admitted.
- **Date** of admission.
- An opinion as to whether the disease or poisoning from which the patient is, or is suspected to be, suffering from **was contracted in hospital.**

The purpose of this requirement is to:

- Identify the responsible **organism**.
- Identify the **source** and **mode** of spread of the infection.
- Identify **carriers**.
- Identify **contacts**.
- **Control** the spread of the disease by appropriate means.

According to the seriousness of the threat to the community, certain diseases are required to be notified immediately by telephone to the 'proper officer', e.g. suspicion of typhoid fever. Further powers under the regulations provide compulsory examination of those suspected of suffering from, or being 'carriers' of, the notifiable disease.

It is an offence in Scotland to send a child to school with a notifiable infectious disease.

Environmental Health Officers are widely involved with disease prevention and control. The Medical Officer is responsible for ensuring necessary procedures are carried out and that all authorities liaise with and take advice from the Chief Medical Officer of Health at the Department of Health. Liaison with the various International Centres for Communicable Disease Control and the World Health Organisation helps to ensure the pattern of disease is monitored and pandemics (world-wide epidemics) are anticipated, prevented, controlled and monitored.

It should be noted that sexually-transmitted diseases, e.g. HIV, AIDS and gonorrhoea, are not normally reportable. This is because it is feared that people would be inhibited from seeking treatment. However, there are various measures which can be taken if there is **imminent danger** to the public.

It is essential that necessary **reporting** is carried out; practice staff may be involved in ensuring that certificates are despatched to the appropriate person in the area. Those persons attending surgery who have **recently returned from abroad** and are complaining of illness should be **isolated** in order to ensure other patients are not **exposed** to infectious illness. Similarly, patients who appear to have skin rashes due to infectious disease should be **separated** from others in the waiting room until they are seen by the doctor and a **diagnosis** is made.

ABBREVIATIONS

BCG	bacillus Camille-Guérin – vaccine against tuberculosis
DT	diphtheria, tetanus – vaccine
DTP	diphtheria, tetanus, pertussis (whooping cough) – vaccine against the three diseases
Hep A	hepatitis A viral infection (water-borne)
Hep B	hepatitis B viral infection (body fluids), also known as serum hepatitis
Hep C	hepatitis C viral infection
Hep non A **Hep non B** **Hep non C**	hepatitis caused by virus other than A, B or C. These are now recognised as D and E.
Hib	*Haemophilus influenzae* bacillus – immunisation for babies against meningitis caused by an organism
MMR	measles, mumps, rubella – vaccine against the three diseases
Td	low-dose diphtheria vaccine

N.B. Hib is now usually combined with DTP vaccine or DT

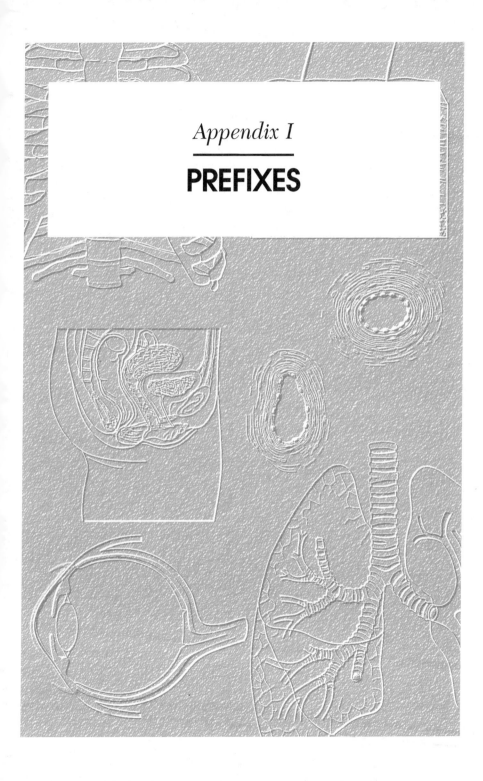

Appendix I

PREFIXES

PREFIXES

PREFIX	MEANING
a-	absence of
ab-	away from
acou-	hearing
acro-	extremities
actino-	ray/sun
ad-	towards
aero-	air
af-	towards/near
agora-	open space
albumen-/albumin-	albumin
amblyo-	dim/dull
amylo-	starch
an-	absence of
ana-	up/excessive
aniso-	equal
ankylo-	crooked/bent
ante-	before
anti-	against
apo-	away from
aqua-	water
athero-	plaque lining blood vessels/porridge
audio-	hearing
auto-	self
baso-	basic
bi-	two
bin-	double/two
blasto-	immature/germ cell
brady-	slow
cata-	down
centi-	a hundredth
chemo-	chemical
chole-	bile
chromo-/ chromato-	colour
circum-	around
co-/con-	together/joined
contra-	against
cor-/coreo-	pupil
cryo-	cold
crypto-	hidden
de-	away, from/removing
deca-	ten
deci-	tenth
demi-	half
dextra-	to the right
di-	two
dia-	through
diplo-	double
dis-	against/separation
disto-	far
dorso-	dorsal (back)
dys-	difficult/abnormal/painful
ec-	out of/away from
ecto-	external/outside/without
electro-	electricity
em-	in
embolo-	plug
en-/endo-	within/in/into
ent-	within
epi-	upon/above/on
ery-	red
eu-	well/good/normal
ex-/exo-	out of/away from
extra-	outside
ferri-/ferro-	iron
flav-	yellow
fore-	before/in front of
galacto-	milk
glyco-	sugar
hecta-	one hundred
hemi-	half
hetero-	unlike/dissimilar
hexa-	six
hidro-	perspiration
homeo-	like
homo-	same
hydro-	water
hygro-	moisture
hyper-	above/high/in excess of normal
hypo-	low/below/under/less than normal
ichthyo-	dry/scaly
idio-	peculiar to individual/own
immuno-	immunity
in-	not/into/within
infra-	below
inter-	between
intra-	within/inside
intro-	inward
iso-	equal
juxta-	next to
kalo-	potassium
kilo-	one thousand
koilo-	spoon
kypho-	crooked/humped/rounded
lacto-	milk
latero-	side
leavo-	left

lepto-	thin/soft	proximo-	near
leuco-/leuko-	white	pseudo-	false
lipo-	fat	psycho-	mind
lordo-	bent forward	pyo-	pus
macro-	large	pyro-	fever
mal-	poor/abnormal	quadri-	four
mano-	pressure	quinqu-	five
medi-	middle	radio-	radiation
mega-/megalo-	big/enlarged	re-	again/back
melano-	black/dark/pigment	retro-	backwards
meso-	middle	saccharo-	sugar
meta-	after/beyond	sapro-	dead/decayed
micro-	small/one-millionth	sarco-	flesh
milli-	thousandth	sclero-	hard
mio-	smaller	scolio-	crooked
mono-	one/single	scota-	darkness
morpho-	form/dream	semi-	half
multi-	many	sero-	serum
myc-	fungus	sex-	six
narco-	deep sleep/stupor	socio-	sociology
natro-	sodium	sono-	sound
necro-	death	spiro-	breath
neo-	new	squamo-	scaly
nocto-	night	staphylo-	grapes/cluster
nulli-	none	steato-	fat
nycto-	night	steno-	narrow
oct-	eight	strepto-	chain
oligo-	scanty/deficiency	sub-	below
onco-	tumour	super-/	
opistho-	backwards	supra-	above
ortho-	straight	syn-	with/together/union
pachy-	thick	syringo-	cavity/tube
paedo-	child	tachy-	rapid/fast
pan-	all	tact-	touching
para-	alongside	ter-	three
patho-	disease	tetra-	four
penta-	five	thermo-	heat
per-	through/by	thrombo-	blood clot
peri-	around	tox-/toxico-	poison
pharmaco-	drug	trans-	across/through
photo-	light	tri-	three
pluri-	many	tropho-	nourishment
pneumo-/		ultra-	beyond
pneumono-	air/gas/lung	uni-	one
polio-	grey	uro-	urine
poly-	many	uvulo-	uvula
post-	after	vaso-	vessel
pre-/pro-	before	ventro-	front/anterior
presbyo-	old age	xantho-	yellow
proto-	first	xero-	dry

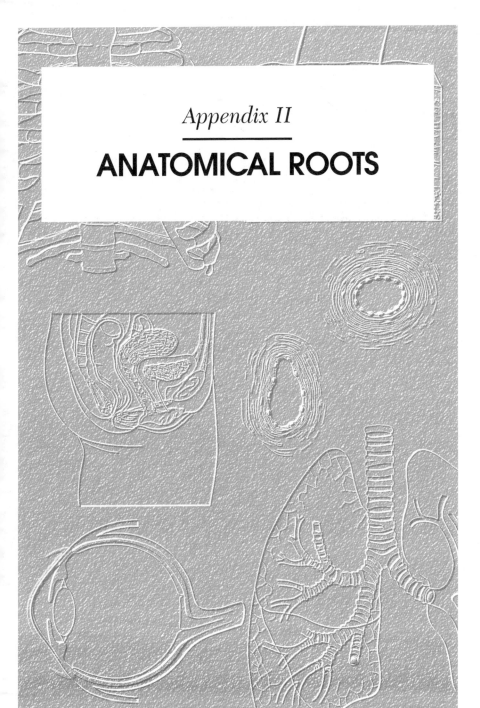

Appendix II

ANATOMICAL ROOTS

ANATOMICAL ROOTS

ANATOMICAL ROOT	MEANING
abdomino-	abdomen
adeno-	gland (any)
adreno-	adrenal gland
alveolo-	air sac
ano-	anus
andro-	man
angio-	vessel
antro-	antrum
aorto-	aorta
appendico-	appendix
arthro-	joint
atrio-	atrium (upper chamber of heart)
axillo-	axilla (armpit)
balano-	penis
blenno-	mucus
blepharo-	eyelid
brachio-	arm
broncho-	bronchus
bronchiolo-	bronchiole
bucco-	cheek
caeco-	caecum
cardio-	heart
carpo-	wrist
cephalo-	head
cerebello-	part of brain (cerebellum)
cerebro-	brain
cervico-	cervix/neck
cheil-	lip
cheiro-	hand
choroido-	choroid (layer of eye)
cholecysto-	gallbladder
choledocho-	common bile duct
chondro-	cartilage
colo-/colono-	colon (large intestine)
coro-	pupil/dermis
corono-	heart
corporo-	body
costo-	rib
cranio-	skull containing brain
culdo-	recto-uterine sac (Pouch of Douglas)
cyclo-	ciliary body (of eye)
cysto-	bladder
cyto-	cell
dacryo-	tear/tear duct
dactyl-	finger
dento-	tooth
derm- / dermato-	skin
digit-	finger/toe
duodeno-	duodenum (part of intestine)
endocardio-	lining of heart
endometrio-	endometrium (lining of uterus)
entero-	intestine
epiglotto-	epiglottis
faci-	face/surface
feto-/foeto-	fetus
gastro-	stomach
genito-	genital
gingivo-	gums
glosso-	tongue
gnatho-	jaw
gyno- / gynaeco-	woman
haemo- / haemato-	blood
hallux-	great toe
hep-/hepato-	liver
histo-	tissue
hystero-	womb
ileo-	ileum (part of intestine)
ilio-	ilium
irido-	iris (of eye)
ischio-	ischium (part of hip bone)
jejuno-	jejunum (part of intestine)
karyo-	nucleus
kerato-	cornea/skin
labyrintho-	labyrinth (part of ear)
lacrimo- / lachrymo- / lacrymo-	tear
lamino-	lamina (part of vertebra)
laparo-	abdomen
laryngo-	larynx
linguo-	tongue
lobo-	lobe
lympho-	lymphatic, lymph
lymphadeno-	lymph gland
lymphangio-	lymph vessel
mammo- / masto-	breast
mastoido-	mastoid (part of ear)
meningo-	meninges
menisco-	meniscus (knee cartilage)
metro-	womb
myco- / myceto-	fungus
myelo-	marrow/spinal cord
myo-/myos-	muscle

myocardio-	myocardium (heart muscle)	recto-	rectum
myometrio-	myometrium (muscle of uterus)	ren-	kidney
		retino-	retina
myringo-	ear drum	rhino-	nose
myxo-	mucous membrane	sacro-	sacrum
naso-	nose	salpingo-	fallopian/uterine tube
nephro-	kidney	sanguino-	blood
nucleo-	nucleus	sarco-	flesh
oculo-	eye	sero-	serum
odonto-	tooth	sialo-	salivary gland
onycho-	nail	sigmoido-	sigmoid colon
oesophago-	oesophagus (gullet)	sino-	space/sinus
oestro-	oestrogen	somato-	body
oo-	egg/ovum	splancho-	viscera/organs
oophoro-	ovary	spermato-	spermatazoa/semen
ophthalmo-	eye	sphygmo-	pulse
opto-	sight	spleno-	spleen
orchio- ⎫	testis	spondylo-	vertebra
orchido- ⎭		stetho-	chest
oro-	mouth	stoma- ⎫	mouth
os-	bone/mouth	stomato- ⎭	
ossic- ⎫	ossicles (bones)	tabo-	tabes
ossiculo- ⎭		tarso-	foot/eyelid
osteo-	bone	tendino-/teno-	tendon
oto-	ear	thelo-	nipples
ovari-	ovary	thoraco- ⎫	chest/thorax
paroto-	parotid gland	thoracico- ⎭	
paedo-	child	thrombo-	blood clot
ped-	foot	thymo-	thymus gland
pericardio-	outer layer of heart (covering of heart)	thyro-	thyroid
		tibio-	tibia
		tilo-	breast
perineo-	perineum	tonsillo-	tonsills
peritoneo-	peritoneum	tracheo-	windpipe/trachea
phako-	lens	tricho-	hair
phallo-	penis	tympano-	ear drum
pharyngo-	pharynx	uretero-	ureter
phlebo-	vein	urethro-	urethra
phono-	voice	uro-	urine/urinary organs
phreno-	diaphragm/mind	utero-	womb
pilo-	hair	uveo-	uveal tract (part of eye)
pleuro-	lung	valvo- ⎫	valve
pneumo- ⎫	lung	valvulo- ⎭	
pneumono- ⎭		varico-	varicose veins
podo-	foot	vasculo-	blood vessel
pollex-	thumb	vaso-	vessel
procto-	anus/rectum	veno-	vein
ptyalo-	saliva	ventrico- ⎫	ventricle (lower chamber of heart)
pyelo-	pelvis of the kidney	ventriculo- ⎭	
pyloro-	pylorus of the stomach	vesico-	vesicle/bladder
prostato-	prostate gland	vestibulo-	vestible of inner ear
rachio-	spine	volo-	palm
radiculo-	nerve root	zoo-	animal

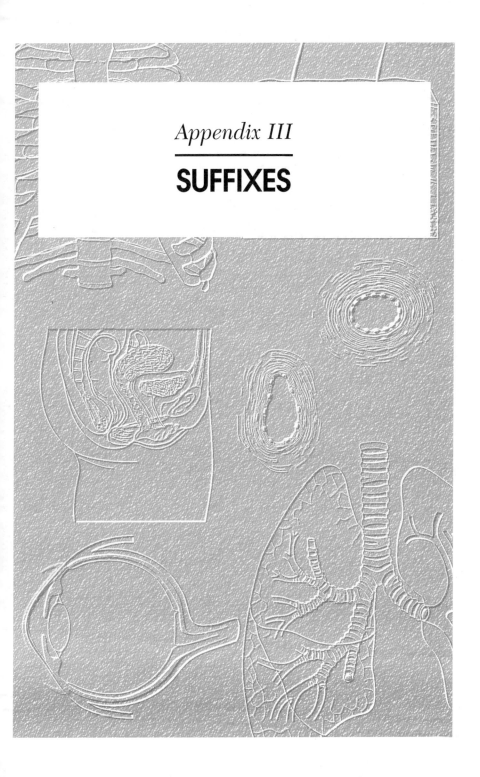

Appendix III

SUFFIXES

SUFFIXES

SUFFIX	MEANING
-a	condition of
-aemia	blood
-ad	towards
-aesthesia	feeling/sensibility
-al	concerning/pertaining to
-algia	pain
-an	concerning/pertaining to
-ase	enzyme
-ate	a salt
-blast	immature cell
-cele	swelling/protrusion
-centesis	to puncture/tapping
-cide	kill/destroy
-cision	cutting
-clasis	destruction of/breaking
-clysis	injection/infusion
-coccus	round cell, type of bacteria
-cyte	cell
-derm	skin
-desis	binding together
-dipsia	thirst
-dynia	pain
-ectasis	dilatation
-ectomy	surgical removal of
-form	having the formation or shape of
-fuge	expelling
-gen	producing/forming
-genesis	forming or origin
-genic	producing or forming
-gogue	increasing flow
-gram	picture/tracing
-graph	machine that records/tracing
-graphy	procedure of recording/tracing
-gravid -gravida	pregnancy
-ia -iasis	condition of/state of
-iatric	pertaining to medicine/physician
-ic	concerning/pertaining to
-iosis -ism	condition of/state of
-itis	inflammation of
-kinesis	movement/activity
-lalia	speech
-lith	stone
-lithesis	slipping
-lithiasis	condition/presence of stones
-lysis	destruction/splitting/breaking down
-malacia	softening
-megaly	enlargement of
-meter	measure
-oedema	swelling caused by excess fluid
-oid	likeness/resemblance
-ology	study of/science of
-oma	tumour
-opia -opsia	condition of the eye (vision)
-oscopy	examination with a lighted instrument
-ose	sugar
-osis	condition of
-ostomy	artificial opening into
-otomy	cutting into/dividing/incision
-ous	like/similar to
-para	given birth
-paresis	weakness
-pathy	disease
-penia	lack of/decreased
-pexy	fixation of
-phage	eating/ingesting
-phagia	swallowing
-phakia	lens (of the eye)
-phasia	speech
-philia	liking/loving/affinity for
-phobia	irrational fear
-phylaxis	protection/prevention
-plasty	form/mould/reconstruct
-plegia	paralysis
-pnoea	breathing
-poiesis	making/production
-ptosis	drooping/falling
-ptysis	cough
-rhythmia	rhythm
-rrhage -rrhagia	burst forth/heavy bleeding
-rrhaphy	sew/repair
-rrhexis	rupture/break
-rrhoea	flow/discharge
-sclerosis	hardening

-scope	lighted instrument used to examine	-stenosis	narrowing
-scopy	examination with a lighted instrument	-sthenia	strength
		-taxia	co-ordination/order
-scotoma	blind spot	-tocia	labour/birth
-somatic	pertaining to the body	-tome	cutting instrument
-sonic	sound	-tripsy	crushing
-spadia	to draw out	-triptor	instrument used to crush
-stasis	cessation of movement/flow	-trophy	nourishment/food
-stat	an agent to prevent moving or change	-tropic	affinity/turning toward
		-tussis	cough
-staxis	dripping (blood)/continuous slight loss	-uria	condition

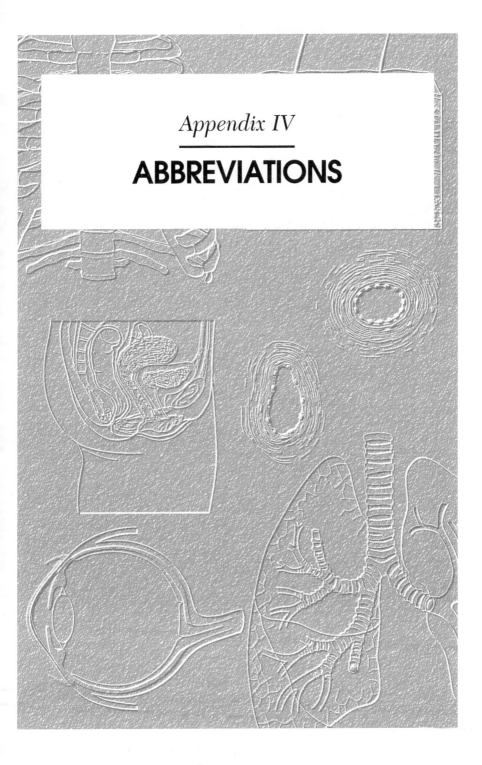

Appendix IV

ABBREVIATIONS

ABBREVIATIONS
Degrees, qualifications, titles and awards

BA	Bachelor of Arts
BAO	Bachelor of the Art of Obstetrics
BC BCh BChir	Bachelor of Surgery
BM	Bachelor of Medicine
BS	Bachelor of Surgery
BSc	Bachelor of Science
CCDC	Consultant in Communicable Disease Control
ChB CChir	Bachelor of Surgery
CM ChM	Master of Surgery
CPH	Certificate in Public Health
CPN	Community Psychiatric Nurse
DA	Diploma in Anaesthetics
DCH	Diploma in Child Health
DCh	Doctor of Surgery
DCP	Diploma in Clinical Pathology
DDS	Doctor of Dental Surgery
DHyg	Doctor of Hygiene
DIH	Diploma in Industrial Health
DLO	Diploma in Laryngology and Otology
DN	District Nurse
Dip Med Rehab	Diploma in Medical Rehabilitation
DM	Doctor of Medicine
DMR	Diploma in Medical Radiology
DO	Diploma in Ophthalmology
DObstRCOG	Diploma in Obstetrics of the Royal College of Obstetricians and Gynaecologists
DOMS	Diploma in Ophthalmological Medicine and Surgery
DPH	Diploma in Public Health
DPM	Diploma in Psychological Medicine
DR	Diploma in Radiology
DSc	Doctor of Science
DTH	Diploma in Tropical Hygiene
DTM	Diploma in Tropical Medicine
FAMS	Fellow of the Association of Managers, Medical Secretaries, Practice Administrators and Receptionists
FDS	Fellow of Dental Surgery
FFARCS	Fellow of Faculty of Anaesthetists, Royal College of Surgeons
FFHom	Fellow of Faculty of Homeopathy
FFR	Fellow of the Faculty of Radiologists
FRCGP	Fellow of the Royal College of General Practitioners
FRCOG	Fellow of the Royal College of Obstetricians and Gynaecologists
FRCP	Fellow of the Royal College of Physicians (London)
FRCPE FRCPEd° FRCPEdin°	Fellow of the Royal College of Physicians of Edinburgh
FRCPS	Fellow of the Royal College of Physicians and Surgeons
FRCPath	Fellow of the Royal College of Pathologists
FRCPsych	Fellow of the Royal College of Psychiatrists
FRCS	Fellow of the Royal College of Surgeons (England)

FRCSE°	Fellow of the Royal College of Surgeons of Edinburgh	**MFHom**	Member of the Faculty of Homeopathy
FRIPHH	Fellow of the Royal Institute of Public Health and Hygiene	**MHyg**	Master of Hygiene
		MMSA	Master of Midwifery of Society of Apothecaries
FRS	Fellow of the Royal Society	**MPH**	Master of Public Health
HVCert	Health Visitors Certificate	**MRCGP**	Member of the Royal College of General Practitioners
LAH	Licentiate of Apothecaries Hall (Dublin)	**MRCOG**	Member of the Royal College of Obstetricians and Gynaecologists
LDS	Licentiate in Dental Surgery		
LM	Licentiate in Midwifery	**MRCP**	Member of the Royal College of Physicians (London)
LRCP	Licentiate of Royal College of Physicians		
LSA	Licentiate of Society of Apothecaries	**MRCPath**	Member of the Royal College of Pathologists
MA	Master of Arts		
MAO	Master of the Art of Obstetrics	**MRCPsych**	Member of the Royal College of Psychiatrists
MAMGP	Member of the Association of Managers in General Practice	**MRCS**	Member of the Royal College of Surgeons (England)
MAMS	Member of the Association of Medical Secretaries, Practice Managers Administrators and Receptionists	**MS**	Master of Surgery
		MSc	Master of Science
		MSW	Medical Social Worker
		OT	Occupational Therapist
MB	Bachelor of Medicine	**PhD**	Doctor of Philosophy
MCh	Master of Surgery	**RGN**	Registered General Nurse
MChD	Master of Dental Surgery	**RN**	Registered Nurse
MChir	Master of Surgery	**SEN**	State Enrolled Nurse (old title)
MChOrth	Master of Orthopaedic Surgery	**SCM**	State Certified Midwife
MCPath	Member of College of Pathology	**SRN**	State Registered Nurse (old title)
MCPS	Member of College of Physicians and Surgeons	**SRP**	State Registered Physiotherapist
MD	Doctor of Medicine		
MDS	Master of Dental Surgery		
MFCP	Member of the Faculty of Community Physicians		

° It is correct to put the initial of the appropriate college after MRCS or FRCS, or LRCP and FRCP for the Royal Colleges of Scotland

Organisations and institutions associated with medical practice

AMGP	Association of Managers in General Practice
AMSPAR	Association of Medical Secretaries, Practice Managers, Administrators and Receptionists
BMA	British Medical Association
BMJ	British Medical Journal
BRCS	British Red Cross Society
CHC	Community Health Council
CHI	Commision for Health Improvement
CMB	Central Midwives Board
DoH	Department of Health
DSS	Department of Social Security
FPA	Family Planning Association
GMC	General Medical Council
GMSC	General Medical Services Committee
HA	Health Authority
HCHS	Hospital and Commuity Health Services
IHSM	Institute of Health Service Managers
LMC	Local Medical Committee
LMG	Local Medical Group
MAAG	Medical Audit Advisory Group
MASTA	Medical Advisory Service for Travellers Abroad
MDU	Medical Defence Union
MPS	Medical Protection Society
MRC	Medical Research Council
NAHAT	National Association of Health Authorities and Trusts
NBTS	National Blood Transfusion Service
NHS	National Health Service
NICE	National Institute of Clinical Excellence
PCG	Primary Care Groups
RCGP	Royal College of General Practitioners
RCN	Royal College of Nursing
RHE	Regional Health Executive
UKCC	United Kingdom Central Council for Nursing Midwifery and Health Visiting
WHO	World Health Organisation

General Medical

ab	abortion
A&E	accident and emergency
A&W	alive and well
ABC	aspiration, biopsy, cytology
abd	abdomen/abdominal
ABR	auditory brain stem response
Acc	accommodation
ACTH	adrenocorticotropic hormone
ad	auris dextra (right ear)
ADD	attention deficit disorder
ADH	antidiuretic hormone
AET/aet	aged
AFP	alpha-fetoprotein (test for abnormality in fetus in amniotic fluid or maternal blood)
AGN	acute glomerulonephritis
AHF	antihaemophilic factor
AI	artificial insemination
AID	artificial insemination by donor
AIDS	acquired immunodeficiency syndrome
AIH	artificial insemination by husband
ALL	acute lymphocytic leukaemia

ALS	amyotrophic lateral sclerosis	CABG	coronary artery bypass graft
AML	acute myeloid leukaemia	CABS	coronary artery bypass surgery
AN	antenatal	CAD	coronary artery disease
ANS	autonomic nervous system	CAPD	continuous ambulatory peritoneal dialysis
AP	artificial pneumothorax	CAT scan } Ct }	computerised axial tomography (X-ray of layers of tissues)
AP&L	anterior, posterior and lateral	CCF	congestive cardiac failure
APH	antepartum haemorrhage	CCU	coronary care unit
APT	activated prothrombin time	CDH	congenital dislocation of the hip
APTT	activated partial thromboplastin time	CHF	congestive heart failure
ARM	artificial rupture of membranes	CIN	cervical intra-epithelial neoplasia
AS	aortic stenosis	CJD	Creutzfeldt–Jacob disease
as	auris sinistra (left ear)		
ASD	atrial septal defect	CLL	chronic lymphocytic leukaemia
ASHD	arteriosclerotic heart disease	CML	chronic myeloid leukaemia
AST	aspartate transaminase (cardiac enzyme)	CNS	central nervous system
Ast	astigmatism	CO	carbon monoxide
au	aures unitas (both ears) or auris uterque (each ear)	C/O	complains of
		CO₂	carbon dioxide
BaE	barium enema	COAD	chronic obstructive airway disease
BaM	barium meal		
BBA	born before arrival	COC	combined oral contraceptive pill
BI	bone injury		
BID	brought in dead	COLD	chronic obstructive lung disease
BM	bowel movement		
BNO	bladder neck obstruction	COPD	chronic obstructive pulmonary disease
BO	bowels open		
BP	blood pressure	CPK	creatine phosphokinase (cardiac enzyme)
BS	breath sounds		
BSE	bovine spongiform encephalopathy ('mad cow' disease)	CPR	cardiopulmonary resuscitation
BSO	bilateral salpingo-oophorectomy	CPT	carpal tunnel syndrome
BUN	blood urea nitrogen	CSF	cerebrospinal fluid
BW	birth weight	CSU	catheter specimen of urine
Bx	biopsy		
C&S	culture and sensitivity	CVA	cerebrovascular accident (stroke)
C1, C2, etc	cervical vertebrae		
CA	chronological age	CVP	central venous pressure
Ca	carcinoma/calcium		

CVS	cardiovascular system / chorionic villus sampling (to detect fetal abnormalities)
Cx	cervix (neck of womb)
D	diopter (lens strength)
db	decibel (measurement of hearing)
D&C	dilatation and curettage (scraping out of womb)
D&V	diarrhoea and vomiting
Dec	deceased
DLE	disseminated lupus erythematosus
DNA	did not attend / deoxyribonucleic acid
DNR	do not resuscitate
DOA	dead on arrival
DOB/dob	date of birth
DS	disseminated sclerosis (old term for MS)
DT	delirium tremens
DU	duodenal ulcer
DUB	dysfunctional uterine bleeding
DVT	deep vein thrombosis
Dx	diagnosis
ECG	electrocardiogram
ECT	electroconvulsive therapy
EDC	expected date of confinement
EDD	expected date of delivery
EEG	electroencephalogram
EMG	electromyogram
EMU	early morning urine
ENT	ear, nose and throat
EOM	extraocular movement
ERCP	endoscopic retrograde cholangiopancreatography
ERPC	evacuation of retained products of conception
ESL	extracorporeal shock-wave lithotripsy
ESN	educationally subnormal
ESR	erythrocyte sedimentation rate
EUA	examination under anaesthetic
FB	foreign body
FBC	full blood count
FBS	fasting blood sugar
FH	family history / fetal heart
FHH	fetal heart heard
FHNH	fetal heart not heard
FMF	fetal movement felt
FNA	fine needle aspiration
FSH	follicle-stimulating hormone
G&A	gas and air
GA	general anaesthetic
GH	growth hormone
GI	gastrointestinal
GOK	God only knows
GOT	glutamicoxalo-acetic transaminase (cardiac enzyme)
GPI	general paralysis of the insane
GTT	glucose tolerance test (to diagnose diabetes mellitus)
GU	genitourinary / gastric ulcer
Hb	haemoglobin (pigmented protein which carries oxygen)
HbA₁ / HBA₁	blood test for diabetes
HCl	hydrochloric acid
HDL	high-density lipoprotein
HDU	high dependency unit
HI	hypodermic injection
HIV	human immunodeficiency virus
HM	hand movement
HNPU	has not passed urine
Hp	*helicobacter pylori*
HPL	human placental lactogen (assay blood test which monitors health of placenta and fetus)
HPU	has passed urine
HPV	human papilloma virus
HRT	hormone replacement therapy
HS	heart sounds
HSV	herpes simplex virus

HVS	high vaginal swab	LFT	liver function test (to diagnose liver disease)
Hx	history	LH	luteinising hormone
ia	intra-articular (into a joint)	LIF	left iliac fossa
ICU	intensive care unit	LIH	left inguinal hernia
IDDM	insulin-dependent diabetes mellitus	LLQ	left lower quadrant
		LMP	last menstrual period
Ig	immunoglobulin	LOA	left occipitoanterior
IM/im	intramuscular	LOL	left occipitolateral
INR	international nor-malised ratio (prothrombin time)	LOP	left occipitoposterior
		LRTI	lower respiratory tract infection
IOFB	intraocular foreign body	LSCS	lower segment cae-sarean section
IOP	intraocular pressure	LTH	luteotropic hormone (prolactin)
IP	inpatient		
IPPB	intermittent positive pressure breathing	LUQ	left upper quadrant
		MA	mental age
IQ	intelligence quotient	MAOI	monoamine oxidase inhibitor (antidepres-sant)
ISQ	in status quo (no change)		
ITU	intensive therapy unit	MC&S	microscopy, culture and sensitivity
IU or U	international unit		
IUC	idiopathic ulcerative colitis	MCH	mean corpuscular haemoglobin
IUCD	intra-uterine contra-ceptive device	MCHC	mean corpuscular haemoglobin concen-tration
IUD	intra-uterine device or intra-uterine death		
IUFB	intra-uterine foreign body	MCV	mean corpuscular vol-ume (size of cell)
		mmol	millimole
IV/iv	intravenous	MND	motor neurone dis-ease
IVC	intravenous cholan-giography		
		MRI	magnetic resonance imaging
IVF	*in vitro* fertilisation	MRSA	multiple-/methicillin-resistant *Staphylococcus aureus*
IVP	intravenous pyelogram		
IVU	intravenous urogram		
K	potassium	MS	multiple sclerosis
KUB	kidney, ureter, and bladder (X-ray)	MSH	melanocyte-stimulat-ing hormone
L&D	light and dark (perceived)	MSU	midstream specimen of urine
L1, L2, etc	lumbar vertebrae	Na	sodium
LA	local anaesthetic	N&V	nausea and vomiting
LCS	left convergent squint (eye turns inwards)	NAD	no abnormality detected/demonstrated
LD	lactate dehydrogenase (cardiac enzyme)	NAI	non-accidental injury
		NBI	no bone injury
LDL	low-density lipoprotein	ND	normal delivery
		NFR	not for resuscitation
LDS	left divergent squint (eye turns outwards)	NG }	new growth nasogastric (tube)

NIDDM	non-insulin-dependent diabetes mellitus	**PMH**	past medical history
nmol	nanomole	**PMS**	premenstrual syndrome
NMR	nuclear magnetic resonance (MRI)	**PN**	postnatal
NOAD	no other abnormality detected	**PNC**	postnatal clinic
NSAID	non-steroidal anti-inflammatory drug	**PND** }	paroxysmal nocturnal dyspnoea / post-nasal drip
nvCJD	new variant Creutzfeldt–Jacob disease (human BSE)	**POD**	pouch of Douglas (retro-uterine fold of peritoneum lying behind the womb)
O_2	oxygen		
OA }	on arrival / osteoarthritis	**POP** }	plaster of Paris / progestogen only pill (contraceptive)
OCD	obsessive–compulsive disorder	**PP** }	placenta praevia / private patient
OD	oculus dexter (right eye)		
OE	on examination	**PPH**	postpartum haemorrhage
OGD	oesophagogastroduodenoscopy	**PR**	per rectum (rectal examination)
OP	outpatient	**PSA**	prostatic-specific antigen (test for cancer of prostate)
OPD	outpatient department		
OS	oculus sinister (left eye)		
OU	oculus uterque (each eye)	**PTCA**	percutaneous transluminal coronary angioplasty
PAP	Papanicolaou smear (cervical smear test)	**PTH**	parathyroid hormone
PAT	paroxysmal atrial tachycardia	**PU**	peptic ulcer
PBI	protein-bound iodine	**PUO**	pyrexia of unknown origin
PCB	post-coital bleeding	**PV**	per vaginam
PCO	patient complains of	**PVC**	premature ventricular contraction
PCP	*Pneumocystis carinii* pneumonia	**RA**	rheumatoid arthritis
PCV	packed cell volume	**RAI**	radioactive iodine
PE	pulmonary embolism	**RAIU**	radioactive iodine uptake
PEFR	peak expiratory flow rate	**RBC**	red blood cell
PERLA/PERRLA	pupils equal (round), react to light and accommodation	**RCS**	right convergent squint (eye turns inwards)
PET }	pre-eclamptic toxaemia / positron emission tomography	**RD** }	respiratory disease / respiratory distress syndrome
pH	acid/alkaline balance	**RDS**	right divergent squint (eye turns outwards)
PH	past history		
PID }	pelvic inflammatory disease / prolapsed intervertebral disc	**REM**	rapid eye movement
		RGP/RP	retrograde pyelogram
		RIF	right iliac fossa
		RIH	right inguinal hernia
PMB	postmenopausal bleeding	**RLQ**	right lower quadrant
		ROA	right occipitoanterior

216

RSI	repetitive strain injury	**T₄**	thyroxine (thyroid hormone)
RT	radiation therapy		
RTA	road traffic accident	**T+**	increased intra-ocular pressure
RUQ	right upper quadrant		
RVS	respiratory virus syndrome	**T-**	decreased intra-ocular pressure
SA	sarcoma	**T&A**	tonsillectomy and adenoidectomy
SADS	seasonal affective disorder syndrome		
SAH	subarachnoid haemorrhage	**TAH**	total abdominal hysterectomy
SB	still birth	**TATT**	tired all the time
SC	*sine correctione* (without correction-spectacles)	**TB**	tuberculosis
SCAN	suspected child abuse or neglect	**TCA** }	to come again tricyclic antidepressant (old type of antidepressant)
SCBU	special care baby unit	**TCI**	to come in
SGOT	serum glutamic oxaloacetic transaminase (liver enzyme)	**TCRE**	transcervical resection of the endometrium
		TENS	transcutaneous electrical nerve stimulation
SGPT	serum glutamic pyruvic transaminase (liver enzyme)		
		THR	total hip replacement
SI }	sexual intercourse international system of units	**TIA**	transient ischaemic attack (in the brain)
		TIBC	total iron-binding capacity
SIDS	sudden infant death syndrome	**TKR**	total knee replacement
SLE	systemic lupus erythematosus		
SMI	school medical inspection	**TLC**	tender loving care
		TLE	temporal lobe epilepsy
SMR	submucous resection	**TMR**	transmyocardial revascularisation
SOB	shortness of breath		
SOL	space-occupying lesion	**TOP**	termination of pregnancy
SSRI	selective serotonin reuptake inhibitor	**tomo**	tomogram
STD	sexually transmitted disease	**TPHA**	*Treponema pallidum* haemagglutination assay (blood test for syphilis)
STYCAR	standard tests for young children and retards (developed by Sheridan to assess visual development)		
		TPR	temperature, pulse and respiration
		TSH	thyroid-stimulating hormone
Sx	surgery, signs and symptoms	**TSS**	toxic shock syndrome
		TTA	to take away
T	tumour	**TUP**	tubal uterine pregnancy
T1, T2, etc }	thoracic vertebrae tumour sizes	**TUR**	transurethral resection (of prostate gland)
T₃	triiodothyronine (thyroid hormone)	**TURB**	transurethral resection of bladder

TURBT	transurethral resection of bladder tumour	**VA**	visual acuity (clarity or accuracy of vision)
TURP	transurethral resection of prostate gland	**VC**	vital capacity
		VCU, VCUG	voiding cystourethrogram
TV	*Trichomonas vaginalis* (infection of vagina causing frothy yellow discharge)	**VF**	visual field
		VI	*virgo intacto* (virgin)
		VSD	ventricular septal defect
TVH	total vaginal hysterectomy	**Vx**	vertex (the crown of the head of the fetus)
U&E	urea and electrolytes	**WBC**	white blood count
UA	urinalysis	**WBC&diff.**	white blood count and different percentages present
UGI	upper gastrointestinal		
µmol	micromole		
UPLD	upper limb disorder	**WRULD**	work-related upper limb disorder
URI	upper respiratory infection		
		XX	female sex chromosomes
URTI	upper respiratory tract infection	**XY**	male sex chromosomes
USS	ultrasound scan		
UTI	urinary tract infection	**YOB**	year of birth

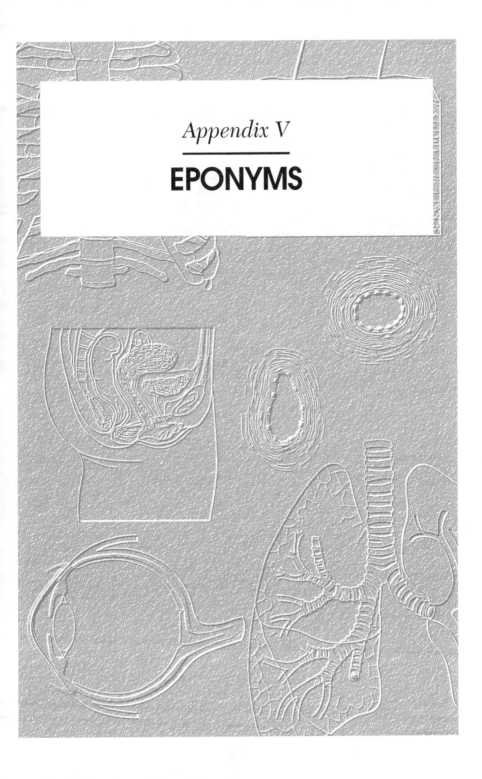

Appendix V

EPONYMS

EPONYMS

The following are a list of diseases, syndromes and tests named after the person or area associated with it.

Addisonian anaemia	pernicious anaemia
Addison's disease	destruction of the adrenal cortex causing deficiency of hormone production
Albee's bone graft	operation of spinal fixation
Albee's operation	producing fixation of hip
Albers-Schonberg disease	a type of osteoporosis ('marble bones')
Allen-Master's sign	pelvic pain resulting from old laceration of broad ligament during childbirth
Alzheimer's disease	early dementia
Argyll Robertson pupils	reacting to accommodation but not to light
Aschoff's nodules	nodules in heart muscle (myocardium) in rheumatism
Babinski's reflex	stroking of the sole of foot causing downward flexion (dorsiflexion)
Bacillus Calmette–Guérin	vaccine for immunisation against tuberculosis
Bankart's operation	treatment of recurrent dislocation of shoulder joint
Banti's syndrome	enlarged spleen in children due to back-pressure of veins, anaemia, jaundice, etc.
Bannwarth's syndrome	neurological manifestation of Lyme disease
Barbados leg	elephant leg
Barlow's disease	infantile scurvy (vitamin C deficiency)
Barret's oesophagus	chronic ulceration of lower oesophagus due to chronic inflammation and epithelial changes
Bartholin's abscess	an abscess of the glands of the vulva
Bell's palsy	one-sided facial paralysis due to pressure on VIIth cranial (facial) nerve
Billroth's operation	partial gastrectomy
Binet's test	IQ intelligence test
Blalock's operation	for correction of Fallot's tetralogy (congenital deformity of the heart)
Boeck's disease	sarcoidosis
Bornholm disease	pain in pleura
Brandt–Andrew's technique	method of delivering the placenta
Braxton Hicks contractions	irregular contractions of uterus occurring after third month of pregnancy
Bright's disease	nephritis
Brodie's abscess	chronic inflammation of the bone marrow (osteomyelitis)
Brudzinski's sign	knee and hip flexion when raising head from pillow
Burkitt's tumour	a form of malignant lymphoma found in African children caused by a virus
Burow's operation	technique for repairing defect of lip
Chadwell-Luc operation	technique for drainage of maxillary antrum (facial sinus)
Charcot's joints	effects of third stages of syphilis or other neurological defect
Charcot's triad	staccato speech, nystagmus (oscillation of eyeballs) and intention tremor in multiple sclerosis
Christmas disease	congenital bleeding disorder due to lack of clotting factor
Chvostek's sign	excessive facial twitching on stimulating facial nerve found in cases of tetanus
Colles' fracture	dinner fork deformity of wrist caused by fracture of lower end of radius
Coombs' test	blood test for antibodies

Creutzfeldt–Jacob disease	degenerative brain disease associated with BSE
Cushing's syndrome	effects of excessive corticosteroid hormones
Da Costa's syndrome	cardiac neurosis (psychological origin of heart symptoms)
Delhi boil	tropical sore
Dengue fever	a viral disease transmitted by mosquitos, occurring in epidemics in tropical and subtropical areas
Derbyshire neck	goitre (enlargement of thyroid gland caused by insufficient iodine in diet)
Dick test	for susceptibility to scarlet fever
Down's syndrome	deformity of chromosome 21 causing mental impairment, enlarged tongue, oval tilted eyes, squint, etc. (formerly known as mongolism)
Duchenne's syndrome	spinal paralysis with polyneuritis
Dupuytren's contraction	painless deformity causing contraction of fingers towards palm
Ebola fever	a haemorrhagic disease
Erb's palsy	deformity of hand causing finger flexion, known as 'waiter's tip paralysis'
Ewing's tumour	sarcoma of shaft of long bone in under 20-year-olds
Fallot's tetralogy	comprising of four congenital heart defects
Felty's syndrome	chronic arthritis associated with leukopenia (deficient number of white blood cells) and enlarged spleen (splenomegaly)
Fothergill's operation	surgical repair of uterine prolapse
Freidreich's ataxia	progressive disease of nervous system resulting in weakness of muscles and staggering
Frölich's syndrome	deficiency of pituitary hormones
Graves' disease	oversecretion of thyroid hormones
Guillain–Barré syndrome	a type of polyneuritis characterised by an ascending paralysis
Gulf War Syndrome	a condition associated with participants in the Gulf War
Hanta virus	a virus causing haemorrhagic disease transmitted by rodents; first identified in USA
Hashimoto's disease	chronic auto-immune disease of the thyroid gland
Haygarth's nodules	swelling of finger joints in arthritis
Henoch's purpura	purple patches caused by bleeding into and from the tissues of the intestinal wall
Hirschsprung's disease	enlarged colon present at birth
Hodgkin's disease	tumour of the lymph glands caused by a virus
Hunter's syndrome	similar to Hurler's syndrome, but less severe
Hurler's syndrome	mental retardation, abnormal development of skeleton, dwarfism, and gargoyle-like facial development due to a metabolic disorder
Huntington's chorea	degenerative genetic disease of the nervous system
Hutchinson's teeth	abnormally notched teeth; part of the signs of congenital syphilis
Jacksonian epilepsy	epilepsy caused by injury or tumour of brain
Kaposi's tumour	pigmented tumour of the skin (common in AIDS)

Kernig's sign	inability to straighten leg at knee joint when thigh is bent at right angles; indicates irritation of meninges
Klinefelter's Syndrome	abnormal chromosome content (47) with XXY chromosomes, causing aggression and sterility
Koch's disease	tuberculosis
Koplik's spots	white spots found in mouth in measles prior to the skin rash occurring; only present in measles
Küntscher nail	used for fixation of fractures of long bones
Kveim test	test for sarcoidosis; intradermal injection followed by later biopsy
Lassa fever	a haemorrhagic disease transmitted by rodents
Legionnaires' disease	acute infection; pneumonia/influenza-type illness caused by *legionella pneumophilia*
Little's disease	spastic paralysis; form of palsy
Ludwig's angina	inflammation of subcutaneous layer of skin of the neck (cellulitis)
Lyme disease	infectious disease caused by ticks, causing widespread neurological and arthritic symptoms
McBurney's point	area on abdomen where pain is felt when testing for appendicitis
Malta fever	undulant fever caused by drinking infected milk (also called brucellosis and Mediterranean fever)
Mantoux test	intradermal test for tuberculosis reaction
Mendel's law	a theory of hereditary

Ménière's disease	disease of inner ear affecting hearing; causes ringing in ears (tinnitus)
Osler's nodules	small painful areas on fingertips in cases of bacterial inflammation of the lining of the heart (endocarditis)
Paget's disease	disease causing brittle bones and cancer of the nipple
Parkinson's disease	progressive disease of the brain producing 'shaking palsy'; treated with L-dopa
Paul–Bunnell test	blood test for glandular fever
Pel–Ebstein fever	recurring fever in Hodgkin's disease
Pott's disease	spinal lesions
Pott's fracture	fracture/dislocation of the ankle
Queckenstedt's test	test performed during lumbar puncture to determine obstruction to flow of cerebrospinal fluid
Ramstedt's operation	surgery to release tight constriction of pyloric sphincter muscle between stomach and duodenum in babies; the condition is congenital
Raynaud's disease	intermittent spasms of arteries supplying extremities
Reiter's syndrome	recurrent urethritis, arthritis, inflammation of the iris, lesions of the mucous membranes, diarrhoea
Rett's syndrome	progressive autism, dementia, etc. associated with metabolic abnormality, principally found in girls
Reye's syndrome	acute disease of brain in young children following a febrile illness (avoid aspirin medication)

Richter's syndrome	a type of lymphoma occurring in the course of chronic leukaemia	**Spitz-Holter valve**	inserted in the brain in hydrocephalus (CNS unable to circulate, causing pressure on brain)
Rinne's test	test for deafness		
Romberg's sign	inability to stand without swaying when eyes are closed and feet placed together	**Still's disease**	a type of arthritis in children
		Stoke–Adam's syndrome	attacks where the heart stops momentarily and loss of consciousness occurs
Rose's test **Rose Waaler** }	blood test for rheumatoid arthritis		
Rovsing's sign	pressure applied to left iliac fossa which causes pain in right iliac fossa (aspirin advised)	**Tay–Sach's disease**	progressive metabolic disease, occurring especially in the Jewish population, causing weakness in muscles and blindness in infancy
Sabin vaccine	live, attenuated (weakened) oral vaccine for poliomyelitis		
Salk vaccine	first vaccine developed using dead organisms (given by injection)	**Tourrette's syndrome**	obsessive–compulsive disorder involving motor and vocal tics
		Turner's syndrome	a congenital disorder in which there are only 45 chromosomes; the missing X chromosome causes dwarfism, etc.
Schick test	determines susceptibility to diphtheria		
Schilling test	special test using radioactive isotopes to determine the levels of vitamin B_{12} in urine (pernicious anaemia)		
		Wasserman test	blood test for syphylis
		Weil's disease	infection caught from the urine of rats; this is the most serious form of leptospirosis
Shirodkar's operation	purse string suture applied to incompetent cervix during pregnancy to prevent miscarriage		
		Widal's test	blood test for typhoid
		Wilms' tumour	malignant tumour of kidney found in young children
Simmonds' disease	anterior pituitary hormone deficiency, usually developed following childbirth when low blood pressure (hypotension) due to haemorrhage has deprived the pituitary gland of its blood supply	**Wilson's syndrome**	disorder causing cirrhosis of liver and widespread jaundice, abnormal metabolism of copper, brain disease, green deposits of pigment in cornea, etc.
		Zollinger–Ellison tumour	tumour of the non-insulin-producing cells of the pancreas
Smith-Peterson nail	used to fix fractures of neck of femur (hip)		

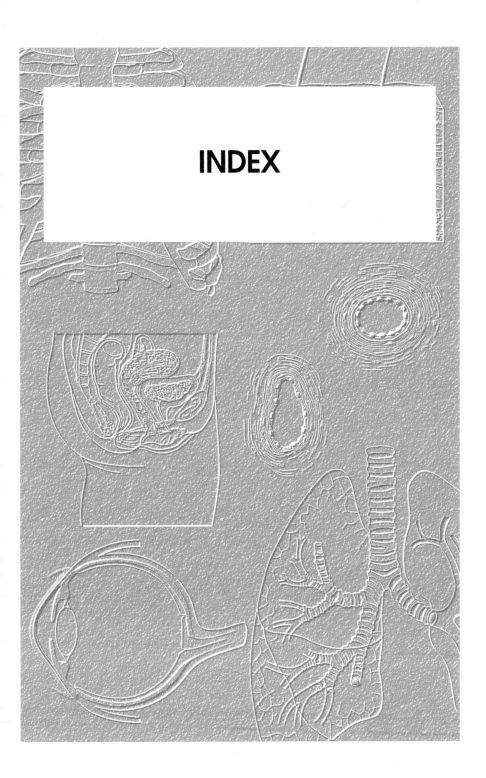

INDEX

flat 19
irregular 19
long 18
sesamoid 19
short 19
bone scan 130
Bowman's capsule 71
brachial artery 174
brain 98–100
brain tumour 174
brainstem 98, 99
   medulla oblongata 99
   midbrain 99
   pons varolii 99
breast 84–85
breast examination 170
bronchi 53
bronchioles 53
buccal cavity 61
bulbourethral glands 94, 95
bundle of His 38
bursa 24

C

calcium 18
calcium metabolism 124
calyx 71
cancellous bone 18
cancer code 171
cancer targets 156
capillaries 40
carbohydrate metabolism 124
cardiac cycle 38
cardiac sphincter 61
cardiopulmonary resuscitation 23, 53
Castle's intrinsic factor 33
CAT scan 129
cauda equina 101
cavities of the body 14
cells 10, 32
central nervous system 98, 129
cerebellum 98, 99, 100
cerebral hemispheres 98
cerebrospinal fluid 100
cerebrum 19, 98–99, 124
   frontal lobe 99
   occipital lobe 99
   parietal lobe 99
   temporal lobe 99
cerumen 113
cervical curvature 23
cervical smears 134, 136, 170
cervix 83

chickenpox 183
child health surveillance 170
childhood diseases 181–3
cholera 186
cholesterol levels 171
chorionic villus sampling 169
choroid 110
chromosomes 10
chronic disease management programmes 157
   asthma 157
   diabetes mellitus 157
chyme 61
ciliary body 110, 113
circumcision 95
clavicle 23, 53
cleft palate 169
click test 170
climacteric 82
clinical waste 137
clitoris 84
clotting 35
club foot 169
cobalt 130
coccyx 22
cochlea 113
colon 61
   ascending 61
   sigmoid 61
   transverse 61
colostrum 85
colour blindness 110
combining vowel 2
Committee on the Safety of Medicines 150
compact bone 18
compatibility 35
computer-enhanced imaging 129
computerised (axial) tomography (CAT) 129
cones 110
congenital dislocation of hip 170
conjunctiva 110
connective tissue 10
consent to immunisation 184
contraindications to immunisation 183
contrast medium 129
controlled drugs 144–145
   prescriptions for 145
cornea 111
coronary heart disease 157
coronary heart disease targets 156
cortex 124
Corti, organ of 113
cortisone 124
costal cartilages 23

cranial nerves 100, 102
cranium 19, 98
cretinism 124
cricoid cartilage 53
criteria for screening 168
CT scan 129
culture medium 135
culture plate 135
curvatures 22–23
  cervical 23
  lumbar 23
  sacral 23
  thoracic 23
Cushing's disease 124
cytology tests 134, 170

D

deamination 62, 70
deglutition 62
dermis 76
desaturation 62
detoxification 62
developmental screening 170
diabetes insipidus 123
diabetes mellitus 71, 124, 157, 171
dialysis 72
diaphragm 26, 53
diastole 42
diastolic pressure 42, 174
digestion 61
diphtheria immunisation 181, 183, 187
disposal of drugs 150
DNA 10
donor 35
  universal 35
Doppler system 130
Down's syndrome 169
dressings and appliances 148
drug abuse/misuse 144
drug addicts 149
DTP immunisation 180
duodenum 61
dura mater 100
dwarfism 123
dyskaryosis 170
dysphagia 62
dysplasia 170

E

ear 113, 114
early morning urine 174, 175
ECG 174
eclampsia 168
EEG 174

efferent nerves 98
ejaculation 95
ejaculatory ducts 95
elderly screening 172
electrocardiography (ECG) 174
  P-wave 174
  QRS complex 174
  T-wave 174
electroencephalography (EEG) 174
endocardium 38
endocrine glands 13, 122
endometrium 83
endoscopy 67
  examples of 67
energy 27
enzymes 61, 62
eosinophils 34
epidemiology 135
epidermal layer 77
epidermis 76
epididymis/epididymides 94, 95
epiglottis 53
epilepsy 174
epithelial tissue 10
eponyms 219–223
ergosterol 77
erythrocytes 32–33
erythropoietin 72
ethmoid sinus 20
eustachian tube 52, 113
evaporation of sweat 77
exchange of gases 54
excretion 12
exocrine glands 12
expiration 23, 53, 54
external ear 113
extrinsic factor 33
eye 110–113
eyeball 110–113
  aqueous humour 110, 111
  choroid 110
  lens 110
  retina 110
  sclera 110
  vitreous humour 110, 112
eyebrows 110
eyelids 110

F

face 20
factor VIII 35
fallopian tubes 82, 83
femoral artery 27

luteinising hormone (LH) 123
luteotrophic hormone 123
lymph 41, 48, 76
lymph capillaries 48
lymph ducts 48, 49
lymph nodes 48, 49
lymph vessels 48
lymphatic system 61
lymphocytes 34–35, 49, 129
lymphoid tissue 124

M

macula 110
magnetic resonance imaging (MRI) 128, 129
malaria 187
malpighian bodies 71
mammary glands 84
mammography 129, 170
mastoiditis 113
maxillary sinus 20
measles immunisation 182
meatus, urethral 72
Medical Control Agency (MCA) 150
Medicines Act 144
medulla 71, 124
medulla oblongata 100
melanin 76
melanin stimulating hormone 123
membranes 13
   mucous 13
   serous 13
   synovial 13
membranous labyrinth 113
menarche 82
meninges 98, 100
   arachnoid mater 100
   dura mater 100
   pia mater 100
meningitis 181
meningococcal meningitis 187
mental illness targets 156
metabolism 12, 124
metastases 49
micro-organisms 135
microbiology tests 135
micturition 72
midbrain 100
middle ear 113
midstream specimen of urine 175
milk 85
mineral salts 12, 32
Misuse of Drugs Act 144
mitral valve 38

MMR immunisation 180
monocytes 35, 49
mons veneris 84
motor area 102
motor nerves 98, 100
movement 12
MRI 128, 129
mucous membranes 13, 76
mumps immunisation 182
murmurs, heart 38
muscle 10, 26
   cardiac 10, 26
   involuntary 10, 26
   voluntary 10, 26
myocardium 38
myometrium 83
myopia 111
myxoedema 124

N

nasal swab 135
naso-pharynx 113
nasolacrimal duct 113
natural immunity 180
needle-stick injuries 137
nephrons 71
neural canal 100
neural-tube defects 169
neutrophils 34
new patient screening 171
newborn screening 169
nipple 84
nitrites 177
non-granular leucocytes 34
nose 52, 114
notifiable diseases 193–196
nuclear medicine 128
nuclear membrane 10, 129
nucleus 10
nurse prescribing 150
nutrition 12

O

occipital lobe 99
oesophagus 27, 60, 61
oestrogen 82, 84, 124
oncology tests 135
ophthalmoscope 110
opportunistic screening 158
optic chiasma 110
optic disc 110
optic fundus 110
optic nerve 110

oral pharynx 61
organ of Corti 113
organs 12
orthoptic exercises 111
osmosis 12, 41
ossicles 113
ossification 18
Otalani's test 170
otitis media 113
'Our Healthier Nation' 154, 158–165
  inequality 159
  key aims 159
  linked programmes 159
  targets 161
ova 82
ovaries 82, 124
oxytocin 84, 123

P

P-wave 174
PACT 149
palate 115
palpation 174
pancreas 62, 124
pancreatic juice 62
Pap test 170
papillae 114
parasympathetic chain 103
parathyroid glands 124
parathyroid hormone (PTH) 124
parietal lobe 99
partial thyroidectomy 124
passive immunity 180
passive smoking 157
pathologists 134
pelvic cavity 14, 24
pelvis 24
pelvis of the kidney 72
penis 94, 95
  foreskin 95
  glans 95
  prepuce 95
pericardium 38
perineum 84
periosteum 18
peripheral nerves 100, 102
peripheral nervous system 98, 102
peristalsis 60, 129
peritoneum 13, 83
pernicious anaemia 33, 61
pertussis immunisation 181
Peyer's patches 49
phagocytes 34

Pharmacy Only Drugs 144
pharynx 52, 115
phenobarbitone 145
phenylketone 169, 177
phlebotomists 134
physiology 10
pia mater 100
pineal body 124
pinna 113
pitressin 123
pituitary gland 82, 84, 122, 124
placenta 84
plasma 32, 134
platelets 32, 35
pleura 13, 53
plexus 100
plurals 6
pneumococcal infections 187
poliomyelitis 180, 182, 183, 187
pons varolii 100
portal circulation 42
positron emission tomography (PET) 129
postnatal care 155
practice formulary 149
prefix 2, 4, 197–199
pregnancy test 174–5
prepuce 95
prescription charges, exemptions 149
prescription only medicines 144
prescription pads 145
prevention 154
  primary 154, 157
  secondary 154, 157
  tertiary 154, 157
primary care groups 154
primary health-care team 154
primary prevention 154, 157
private prescriptions 145, 150
progesterone 82, 84, 124
prolactin 84, 123
prolapse 27
prostate cancer screening 171
prostate gland 94, 95
protein in urine 177
prothrombin 35, 62
protoplasm 10
public health 155
public health laboratory 134
pulmonary artery 39, 41
pulmonary circulation 42
pulmonary valve 38
pulmonary veins 40, 41
pulse 42–43

pupil 110
pyloric sphincter 61

Q

QRS complex 174
quadrants 14

R

rabies 186
radioactive isotopes 128, 129
radiographer 128
radiologist 128
radiotherapist 130
radiotherapy 128
radium 130
reabsorption 71, 72
read codes 154
recall scheme 170
receptionist's role in preventive medicine 158
recipient 35
  universal 35
reflex arc 102
refraction 111
Regional Blood Transfusion Centre 134
regions of the abdomen 14
renal threshold 71
repeat prescriptions 145-148
  collection 149
  computerised 147
  preparation 147
  requests 146
  storage 149
reproduction 12, 82
respiration 12, 54–56
respiratory centre 54
retina 110
Rhesus factor 35, 168
rheumatic fever 38
ribcage 23
risk factor targets 156
rods 110
Röentgen rays 128
root/stem 2, 3–4
  anatomical 201–203
rubella 168
  immunisation 182

S

sacral curvature 23
sacrum 22, 24
saliva 62
salivary glands 62
Schedule one drugs 144

Schedule two drugs 144, 145
Schedule three drugs 144, 145
Schedule four drugs 144
Schedule five drugs 144, 145
schedule, immunisation 180–181
scintigram 130
sclera 110
screening 168–172
  adult 170–171
  antenatal 168–169
  criteria 168
  developmental 170
  elderly 172
  HIV 171
  newborn 169
  new patient 171
  opportunistic 158
  prostate cancer 171
  testicular 171
  triple 169
scrotum/scrota 94
sebaceous glands 76, 77
secondary prevention 154, 157
secretion 71, 72
security of premises 150
semicircular canals 113
seminal fluid 95
seminal vesicles 94, 95
sensitivity 12, 135
sensory nerve endings 76
sensory nerves 98, 100
serology 134
serous membranes 13
serum 32
sesamoid bones 19
sharps 137
short bones 19
sickle-cell anaemia 168, 169
sigmoid colon 61
sinu-atrial node 38
sinuses 20, 52
  ethmoid 20
  frontal 20
  maxillary 20
  sphenoid 20
skeleton 18, 19
  appendicular 19
  axial 19
skin 76–80
skull 19
small intestine 61
  duodenum 61
  ileum 61